Handbook of Human Oocyte Cryopreservation

Handbook of Human Oocyte Cryopreservation

Eleonora Porcu, MD
Director, Infertility and IVF Center, Department of Gynecology, Obstetrics and Pediatrics,
University Hospital S. Orsola-Malpighi, Bologna;
Assistant Professor in Reproductive Medicine, University of Bologna, Italy

Patrizia Maria Ciotti, BSc
Research Scientist, Infertility and IVF Center, University of Bologna, Italy

Stefano Venturoli, MD
Professor, Department of Gynecology, Obstetrics and Pediatrics, University of Bologna, Italy

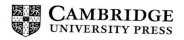

CAMBRIDGE
UNIVERSITY PRESS

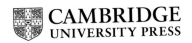

Shaftesbury Road, Cambridge CB2 8EA, United Kingdom

One Liberty Plaza, 20th Floor, New York, NY 10006, USA

477 Williamstown Road, Port Melbourne, VIC 3207, Australia

314–321, 3rd Floor, Plot 3, Splendor Forum, Jasola District Centre, New Delhi – 110025, India

103 Penang Road, #05–06/07, Visioncrest Commercial, Singapore 238467

Cambridge University Press is part of Cambridge University Press & Assessment, a department of the University of Cambridge.

We share the University's mission to contribute to society through the pursuit of education, learning and research at the highest international levels of excellence.

www.cambridge.org
Information on this title: www.cambridge.org/9780521192392

First published 2013

A catalogue record for this publication is available from the British Library

Library of Congress Cataloging-in-Publication data
Porcu, Eleonora.
Handbook of human oocyte cryopreservation / Eleonora Porcu, Patrizia
    Maria Ciotti, Stefano Venturoli.
       p.   ;   cm.
    Includes bibliographical references and index.
ISBN 978-0-521-19239-2 (Hardback)
I. Ciotti, Patrizia M.   II. Venturoli, Stefano.   III. Title.
[DNLM: 1. Cryopreservation–methods.   2. Oocytes–cytology. WQ 205]
570.75´2–dc23

                                                            2012022020

ISBN   978-0-521-19239-2   Hardback

Contents

Contents

Why freeze human eggs? Clinical and biological indications for human oocyte cryopreservation

Ethical and legal indications

In recent years, knowledge of mammal embryo cryobiology has increased considerably. In the human field, embryo cryopreservation has been prompted by the surplus embryos (embryos not immediately used for reproduction) generated during in vitro fertilization programs and embryo transfer (IVF-ET). Since the beginning of extracorporeal fertilization, human embryo freezing has become a requirement demanded by the human fertility therapy procedure. Initially, because of low embryo implant rates, procedures that stimulated many follicles were used to obtain many oocytes and consequently generate many embryos to make up for their lack of vitality. This strategy increased not only pregnancy rates, but also the number of multiple pregnancies and associated complications. Scientific and technological developments led to an improvement in embryonic viability and it was decided to reduce the number of transferred embryos to a maximum of two or three, which is currently the number generally accepted by the scientific community. The generation of an excessive number of embryos gradually appeared unsuitable. The only solution seemed to be that of freezing those in excess, a technique which was successfully attained. However, embryo storage meets with intrinsic ethical reservation on the part of some couples who prefer the number of oocytes for insemination to be reduced to a minimum. Generally speaking, ethical concerns are also present among researchers and the wider public, so much so that, in some countries such as Germany and Italy, this technique has been strongly restricted and sometimes even forbidden.

Apart from ethical reservation, embryo cryopreservation can cause legal issues. Frozen embryos belong equally to the two people who generated them and who may decide, in time, to divorce. In this case, the fate of the embryos is uncertain and will depend on the decision of a court of law. Oocyte freezing would avoid all these ethical and legal problems.

Since the announcement of the first pregnancy from cryopreserved embryos (Trounson and Mohr, 1983), embryo cryopreservation has been widely used and it has accounted for a significant percentage of the treatments of medically assisted procreation. In 2002 the "National Summary of Fertility Centers Report" (NSFCR) reported that 97% of the 391 US infertility clinics offered the opportunity to cryopreserve embryos. About 17% of treatments of medically assisted procreation involve the transfer of frozen embryos. In 2002 more than 400 000 embryos were cryopreserved in the United States. A similar increase in the use of embryo cryopreservation also occurred in Europe and Australia. It was estimated that there were 52 000 frozen embryos in the United Kingdom in 1996, 71 000 frozen embryos were reported in Australia and New Zealand in 2003 (Hoffman et al., 2003) and 15 000 frozen embryos were reported in Canada in 2003 (Newton et al., 2007).

Studies suggest that the storage of surplus embryos is progressively increasing because of the tendency to reduce the number of transferred embryos and the improved success rates of medically assisted procreation techniques. The rapid increase in the use of the cryopreservation method has not allowed us to acquire an adequate awareness of the psychological, social and legal consequences of its use. Moreover, an accurate assessment of the "destiny" of the frozen embryos is necessary because of their progressive increase. There are several choices: the embryos can be used in new in vitro fertilization (IVF) cycles, they can be donated to another infertile couple, they can be used in research or they can be destroyed. The couple can also choose to extend the length of time the embryos remain frozen beyond the deadline, which varies depending on the country.

The great majority of the embryos (88%) are cryopreserved in order to be used in a subsequent cycle. Only 2% of the embryos are cryopreserved in order to be donated to other couples, or they are destroyed (Bankowski et al., 2005). In Klock's (2001) study 107 couples out of 404 (26%) had remaining frozen embryos three years after the treatment and only 17 of those couples were still in treatment. Fifty-two out of 91 couples (57%) responded to the center's analyses: 17 of these 52 (33%) chose to destroy the embryos, 7 (13%) chose to donate to an infertile couple, 5 (10%) to donate to research, 15 (29%) to extend the cryopreservation and 2 (4%) were undecided (Bankowski et al., 2005). Some centers have asked couples to choose the embryo's destiny before IVF treatment to avoid possible unnecessary storage of frozen embryos. These preliminary choices do not take into account the factors which can occur during and after treatment. The validity of a preliminary consensus is questionable because the request is not associated with the inability of the couple to express a consensus at a later time but rather with the organizational needs of the center. The possibility of choice should be provided to the couple. The preliminary consensus should be reserved only for the cases in which one or both spouses are unable to make a decision. The only exception to this rule are cases in which a certain provision concerning the embryos is an essential condition of access to the treatment for one of the two partners (Pennings, 2002; Newton et al., 2007).

Many couples change their minds about the embryo's destiny during treatment. This change is associated with the outcome of the treatment and it confirms the need for a dual informed consensus. In fact in Klock's (2001) study only 12 of 41 couples (29%) confirmed the choice expressed before treatment. Newton et al. (2007) evaluated the changes in the choice of the couples and correlated them with the treatment outcomes. Thirty percent of the examined couples had not used the embryos after five years and 31% of these couples had not updated their provisions about the embryo's destiny. The couples who had achieved a pregnancy were more likely to provide new indications and to choose to destroy the embryos rather than donate them for research. Fifty-nine percent of the couples changed their mind about the destiny of their embryos after the treatment (Table 1.1) (Newton et al., 2007).

These data show that the majority of embryos are destined to never be transferred into the uterus in the absence of a specific legislation for the protection of the embryos. In the United States the majority of people consider an embryo as an inanimate biological entity that cannot enjoy human rights. Therefore a change in US law to modify the legal status of the embryo does not seem realistic. The only federal restriction regards the government support in the creation and destruction of the embryos. The amendment "Dickey-Wicker" forbids the use of federal funds in case of creation, destruction or damage to embryos. The laws change depending on the State: four States regulate the donation of frozen embryos and two States govern their adoption. Among these six, only Louisiana provides protection

Table 1.1. Preferences expressed by couples prior to treatment and the final choice of the destiny of cryopreserved embryos

Options	Number of couples (%)	
	Pretreatment directive	Disposition
Discard	60 (26)	97 (42)
Research	149 (64)	102 (44)
Donation	N/A	18 (8)
Continued storage	N/A	15 (6)
No directive [b]	23 (10)	N/A
Total	232 (100)	232 (100)

N/A = not applicable.
[b] No pretreatment directive obtained.
Reproduced from Newton et al. Changes in patient preferences in the disposal of cryopreserved embryos. Hum Reprod 2007;**22**(12):3124–8 by permission of the European Society of Human Reproduction and Embryology.

for the embryo, while the other States only provide protection for the couples willing to donate or adopt embryos. In fact, only in Louisiana is an embryo considered as a "human being" with the dignity and the rights of a legal person. Therefore, the creation of embryos is only allowed for transferring them to the uterus. However, the majority of States do not have a specific definition of "embryo" and they accept the definition of the High Court of the United States: "the unborn has never been recognized in the law as a person in the whole sense."

The Courts have often considered the embryos like property. In a Tennessee case (1992) a divorced couple asked the court to legislate on the destiny of their frozen embryos because the father wanted to destroy them while the mother wanted to transfer them to her uterus or to donate them to another couple. The trial judge considered the embryo as a human being and supported the transfer of the embryos into the uterus, but the Court of Tennessee changed this decision; they did not consider the embryo as a human being and supported the destruction of the frozen embryos. Similarly in the case Kass vs. Kass (1998) the status of human being of the embryo was denied and the law supported the spouse who wanted to avoid the pregnancy. A similar sentence was issued in 2000 to reject a previously signed agreement giving the custody of the embryos to the wife in case of divorce. In 2003 the Supreme Court of Iowa affirmed that the State only has to take care of the welfare of already born children and not of any fertilized oocytes not yet implanted.

In Europe, various provisions relating to embryo cryopreservation exist. In Germany the "Embryo Protection Act" (1990) states that more than three embryos per cycle of IVF cannot be created and that all embryos must be transferred to the uterus; embryo freezing and destruction are forbidden. The "French Bioethic Law" (1994) forbids embryo production for carrying out research and for obtaining stem cells. A maximum number of embryos which can be created is not established and embryo freezing is not forbidden. Also in Switzerland, there is a law that prohibits the creation of embryos for research purposes in order to protect the legal rights of the human embryos; however, research is allowed on any supernumerary embryos (Brugger, 2009).

Before the present legal regulation, in Italy embryo cryopreservation was carried out in a few centers; in 2003 there were 74 centers (37.4%) offering embryo cryopreservation.

The introduction of the Law 40/2004 reduced significantly the number of embryos stored in the centers. In fact the Law establishes that each IVF treatment must produce no more than three embryos to be transferred into the uterus. In 2000, the number of embryos stored in the assisted reproductive technology (ART) centers was 24 452. In 2007 the Italian National Institute of Health finished the first phase of the count of the abandoned embryos in the centers: only 8 out of 88 surveyed centers affirmed having no frozen embryos stored. Fifty-four (67.5%) centers declared having abandoned frozen embryos while the remaining 26 centers (32.5%) reported having no abandoned frozen embryos. Therefore, in 2007, the total number of abandoned frozen embryos was 3415 belonging to 825 couples.

Since 2003, the number of embryo thawing cycles gradually decreased from 3102 to 704 in 2007, that is 1.6% of the ART cycles in Italy. Instead, the number of oocyte freezing and thawing cycles progressively increased from 102 in 2003 to 2994 in 2007. However, oocyte cryopreservation is still performed in relatively few centers. In 2006 and 2007 the centers that have not performed any oocyte freezing cycles comprised 43.5% and 40.9% of centers, respectively. In 2006 in the Italian centers, 32 860 oocyte pickups were performed and 223 359 oocytes were recovered. The average number of recovered oocytes per cycle was 6.8. Of these only 38.8% were inseminated, 12.9% was cryopreserved, while 107 832 oocytes (48.3%) were rejected. In 2007 the situation was similar: 35 645 oocyte pickups were performed and 234 004 oocytes were recovered (the average was 6.6 oocytes per cycle). Of these 38.3% (89 645 oocytes) were inseminated, with an average of 2.5 oocytes per sample, 11.8% (27 513 oocytes) were cryopreserved (0.8 per cycle) and 49.9% (116 846 oocytes) was rejected (3.3 oocytes per cycle).

In 2009, the High Court of Italy (Act 151/2009) eliminated the prohibition of generating more than three embryos. The new limitation established that the number of produced embryos should be that strictly necessary to be transferred. On the other hand, the High Court did not cancel the prohibition of embryo freezing, except in cases of patient health risks. In actual fact, the interpretation of this rule by a number of ART centers led to a new, huge increase in the number of frozen embryos with potentially uncertain destiny. Therefore, storing eggs instead of embryos should be taken into consideration.

Fertility-saving indications

In the last 30 years, new cancer treatments have improved patient survival rates. The survival rate for all types of tumors is 50%; 90% for Hodgkin's disease, 4–67% for acute lymphocytic leukemia and 33–77% for Wilms' disease diagnosed in childhood. Survival of breast cancer patients has reached 70–75% (National Cancer Institute, 1973–1987). Beyond survival, the quality of a patient's life has now become a key issue. Alterations of reproductive functions in cancer patients depend on both the underlying tumor type and ensuing therapy. It is well known that antiblastic drugs and radiotherapy cause serious damage to the gonads, in many cases inducing premature ovarian failure. Moreover, several studies have shown that the neoplasm itself can reduce fertility (Nieto et al., 1999; Bahadur, 2000). Pal et al. (1988) reported that patients with neoplastic pathologies had lower ovarian quality compared with controls. Although the number of oocytes collected was the same for both groups, oocyte quality, mature oocyte and fertility rates were lower among oncology patients.

Structural and ultrastructural research has shown gonad alterations among patients receiving chemotherapy to be fairly heterogeneous. Derangement depends on patient age; when therapy was started; and the type, dosage and duration of cancer therapy (Nicosia *et al.*, 1984 ; Marcello *et al.*, 1990). Observational evidence indicates that, after chemotherapy, the ovaries of prepubertal adolescents are less affected than those of older patients (Meirow, 2000). In a retrospective study carried out in cooperation with the Rizzoli Orthopaedic Institute of Bologna, similar findings were reported. This study followed the reproductive function of 92 women who had received chemotherapy. Sixty-nine percent of the 92 women had amenorrhea during chemotherapy and 2 of these (all post pubertal at the time of cancer therapy) presented premature ovarian failure (permanent amenorrhea) (Longhi *et al.*, 2000).

Both pharmacological and surgical therapy show significantly increased survival of cancer patients (McVie, 1999); consequently, an increasing number of patients face a life of impaired fertility induced by cancer treatment. Several preventive tools have been proposed to preserve reproductive capacity. Ovarian tissue cryopreservation has been investigated in the past few years as a fertility-saving procedure (Oktay *et al.*, 2004), and the first live birth has been reported after auto-transplantation of ovarian grafts (Donnez *et al.*, 2004). The risk of reintroducing neoplastic cells with this procedure must, however, be kept in mind. On the other hand, in vitro maturation of early immature follicles in tissue presently appears to be not yet reliable (Gook *et al.*, 2004). Oocyte harvesting, fertilization and subsequent embryo storage have also been proposed for partnered women. However, ethical and pragmatic considerations should be taken into account in this choice.

Oocyte storage may be an alternative which does not raise ethical concerns. It might be considered the ideal strategy for preserving the fertility of cancer patients provided they can postpone chemotherapy. This option is feasible in several neoplastic conditions as well as for patients with severe endometriosis and genetic premature ovarian failure. The American Society of Clinical Oncology and the American Society for Reproductive Medicine (ASRM) have issued guidelines recommending that the potential effects of cancer treatment on fertility and the options to preserve fertility should be presented to the patient in the initial stage of treatment (The Ethics Committee of the American Society for Reproductive Medicine, 2005; Lee, 2006).

With heightened public awareness, more aggressive screening and treatment innovation, survival rates for cancer patients are anticipated to increase steadily, allowing more patients to look forward to a normal life after cancer. Unfortunately, radical surgery and chemo- and/or radiotherapy can leave patients infertile or sterile. Goodwin *et al.* (1999) estimated that 53–89% of breast cancer patients treated with chemotherapy undergo premature menopause; the risk for premature menopause was found to be strongly associated with the age of the patient and the use of systemic chemotherapy. In a study of young cancer patients, Meirow (2000) found that the use of alkylating agents, such as cyclophosphamide and busulfan, frequently used in childhood cancer, had an odds ratio (OR) of 4.0 for ovarian failure, which is significantly higher than platinum agents (OR: 1.8), plant alkoids (OR: 1.2) or anti metabolites (OR: <1). The radiation damage is dose-related and depends on fractionation schedule and irradiation field. In women the severity of damage is also influenced by age at the time of exposure to radiotherapy; younger women have, in fact, a greater reserve of primordial follicles than older women and they may thus have a higher remaining primordial pool after a cancer treatment (Wallace *et al.*, 2005).

Table 1.2. Oocyte cryopreservation in patients undergoing antiblastic therapy

Patients	Pathology	Age	Stimulation days	Estradiol	Number of FSH ampoules	Cryopreserved oocytes
1	CML	26	12	450	33	22
2	CML	27	9	1200	30	16
3	Craniopharyngiomas	14	8	750	28	18
4	Medulloblastoma	15	13	630	36	25
5	Myelofibrosis idiopathic	18	12	2820	31	28
6	Essential thrombocytosis	22	11	1150	38	17
7	Hodgkin's disease	17	12	950	36	21
8	CML	24	10	820	29	12
9	Multiple sclerosis	27	10	350	34	17
10	CML	21	9	630	32	12
11	Ewing's sarcoma	16	11	820	33	6
12	Wilms' tumor	19	13	615	39	15
13	CML	14	11	840	37	19
14	Hodgkin's disease	15	11	1230	34	11
15	CML	24	14	780	42	12
16	Ewing's sarcoma	18	13	1200	38	7
17	Hodgkin's disease	23	9	1900	28	9
18	CML	17	12	480	36	12
	Mean ± S.D.	19 ± 4	11 ± 2	978 ± 558	34 ± 4	15 ± 6

CML: chronic myelogenous leukemia.
Reprinted from *Eur J Obstet Gynecol Reprod Biol*, **113**(Suppl 1), Porcu E, Fabbri R, Damiano G, Fratto R, Giunchi S, Venturoli S, Oocyte cryopreservation in oncological patients, S14–16, Copyright 2004, with permission from Elsevier.

Oocyte cryopreservation has become a potentially good option for preserving female fertility, particularly for oncological patients, as was documented for the first time in 2004. Porcu *et al.* (2004) reported data regarding cryopreservation of oocytes from young women who had to undergo cancer treatments. In these young oncological patients, the ovarian stimulation was found to be very efficient, with the retrieval and storage of an average of 15 oocytes per patient that can lead to about two embryo transfers after recovery from the malignancy (Table 1.2).

The first births recently reported demonstrate that oocyte cryopreservation in oncology is a reliable option. Frozen oocytes of a cancer patient were first used in a gestational carrier (Yang *et al.*, 2007), who conceived with frozen oocytes belonging to a patient with Hodgkin's lymphoma that were retrieved and cryopreserved before radiotherapy commenced. Ten out of twelve cryopreserved oocytes survived after thawing and nine were fertilized and developed into good quality embryos, which were transferred in three different cycles to a gestational carrier. A singleton pregnancy was achieved after the third transfer, resulting in the delivery of a healthy male. However, this result was reached thanks to the use of surrogate motherhood, which is not allowed in the majority of countries. Porcu et al. (2008) reported the first pregnancy and delivery from frozen eggs in a cancer patient. After freezing her oocytes, the patient underwent bilateral ovariectomy for ovarian cancer and four years later conceived using her own cryopreserved oocytes, and carried on the pregnancy herself. Seven oocytes were retrieved before ovariectomy. After four years three oocytes were thawed. The survival rate of 100% as well as the fertilization and cleavage rate of 100% demonstrated that eggs may be safely stored for several years. The twin pregnancy progressed uneventfully to term with the birth of healthy twins. The duration of oocyte storage does not seem to interfere with the oocytes' survival as pregnancies occurred even after several years of gametes cryopreservation in liquid nitrogen.

The same group at the University of Bologna has recently obtained the birth of a healthy male from a frozen oocyte of a breast cancer patient. The patient underwent oocyte cryopreservation before chemotherapy for breast cancer. Sixteen oocytes were collected and 14 cryopreserved. After two years and seven months, a cycle of oocyte thawing was performed, with the thawing of four oocytes, all of which survived and were fertilized. Three embryos were transferred into the uterus leading to a single pregnancy that led to the birth of a healthy male at 37 weeks' gestation.

The correct selection of candidates for fertility preservation by oocyte cryopreservation is very important, in order to offer the most suitable and safe technique to each patient. Oocyte cryopreservation is, actually, the best technique for women without a partner, because it does not require surgery and it has already resulted in a significant number of live births, unlike ovarian tissue cryopreservation, which is still an experimental technique. The selection of patients should take into account the age of the women and should include an ovarian reserve assessment by non-invasive methods, such as anti-Mullerian hormone (AMH) and follicle-stimulating hormone (FSH) levels and antral follicles count.

A limit of oocyte cryopreservation is the timing of the procedure; in fact it cannot be proposed to women that must immediately begin chemotherapy because it requires 10–15 days for the ovarian stimulation and oocyte retrieval. Another important issue is the choice of the stimulation protocol, which should take into account the type and stage of the neoplastic disease and the receptor assessment. In cases of estrogen-sensitive tumors the stimulation should be adapted in order to minimize the increase in estrogen levels: this can be achieved by reducing the dose of gonadotropins and by adding aromatase inhibitors to gonadotropins. The most recommended aromatase inhibitor is letrozole at the dose of 5 mg/die, because it shows a good tolerability and a high efficacy in reducing oestradiol levels (Azim et al., 2008; Requena et al., 2008).

An interesting application of oocyte cryopreservation in association with transplant-ation of ovarian cortical tissue in a patient with breast cancer has recently been performed, resulting in the birth of two healthy males. A 36-year-old patient diagnosed with atypical medullar breast cancer underwent a laparoscopic right ovarian cortex extraction before chemotherapy and radiotherapy. The ovarian tissue was cryopreserved using a slow freezing protocol and thawed after two years, when the patient was considered free of disease. The cortical strips were attached to the left ovary that appeared depleted of follicles. Then the patient underwent four different cycles of ovarian stimulation, two of these followed by the vitrification of nine oocytes overall. At warming, all the oocytes survived and seven achieved fertilization; two of these were replaced in the uterus leading to a twin pregnancy (Sànchez-Serrano et al., 2010) (Table 1.3).

An additional strategy to preserve female fertility is oocyte cryopreservation after retrieval of immature oocytes from ovarian tissue, in the absence of previous ovarian stimulation (prior to freezing). This technique can be applied in patients with polycystic ovary syndrome (PCOS), where ovarian stimulation is associated with a significant risk of hyperstimulation syndrome, or in young women without male partners who are affected by malignancies and must begin cytotoxic therapy immediately. The cryopreservation may cover oocytes at the stage of germinal vesicles, or in vitro matured oocytes. In the first case, in vitro maturation (IVM) occurs after the thawing; the cryopreservation of these immature oocytes, which are characterized by widespread chromatin, seems able to prevent depolymerization and, theoretically, reduces the risk of aneuploidy and polyploidy.

Current literature suggests that to obtain a homogeneous cohort of oocytes to mature in vitro, the largest follicular diameter should be 12 mm. Normally the oocytes in this cohort of follicles are all germinal vesicle stage at collection (Smitz et al., 2011). Oocyte maturation is defined as the resumption and completion of the first meiotic division from germinal vesicle stage to metaphase II stage; to achieve competency the fully grown oocyte must undergo nuclear maturation and cytoplasmic differentiation. An efficient IVM protocol must be able to reproduce an environment that will not only sustain oocyte growth but also allow full competence.

The first human oocyte IVM was reported by Edwards (1965). Since this first experiment, the methodology has been refined and considerable progress has been achieved in terms of oocyte maturation and pregnancy rates. In 1988 Mandelbaum obtained, after thawing of frozen oocytes at different maturation stages, the same percentage of morphologically intact oocytes for each maturation stage. In contrast to that observed in guinea pigs, mature human oocyte cryopreservation did not appear clearly correlated with the best morphological characteristics. Sixty percent of immature oocytes resumed meiosis after thawing, and only 8% reached metaphase II (Mandelbaum et al., 1988b). The first successful IVM birth resulted from immature oocytes collected at Cesarean section in an oocyte donation cycle (Cha et al., 1991).

Toth reported an 83.3% (60/72) maturation rate to metaphase II for prophase I oocytes, with a 57.7% fertilization rate and a 3.3% blastocyst rate. According to this study, cryopreserved immature oocytes can resume meiosis after thawing, and reach full maturation, with maturation rates, fertilization and cleavage rate comparable to those of non-cryopreserved oocytes (Toth et al., 1994). This finding was not confirmed in subsequent studies that achieved very low maturation rates and fertilization rates (Son et al., 1996). Park et al. in 1997 sought to provide an explanation for the limited success in terms of fertilization and development, assuming damage to chromosomes and microtubules of immature oocytes. They concluded that in vitro matured oocytes that had previously been cryopreserved showed an increased incidence of chromosomal and microtubular abnormalities (Park et al., 1997). In 1998, Tucker et al. obtained the only birth after germinal vesicle cryopreservation; 3 out of 13 cryopreserved germinal vesicles survived, 2 oocytes had matured and fertilized normally, with the birth of a healthy female (Tucker et al., 1998a).

The overall data published suggest that oocyte cryopresevation should be performed at the mature methaphase II stage, following IVM, rather than at the immature germinal

Table 1.3. Clinical results achieved with oocyte cryopreservation in oncological patients

	Yang, 2007 (first birth in gestational carrier)	Porcu, 2008 (first birth in patient with ovarian cancer)	Sànchez-Serrano, 2010 (birth in breast cancer after transplantation of ovarian tissue)	Porcu, unpublished data, 2012 (birth in patient with breast cancer)
Patient's age	27	26	38	37
Pathology	Hodgkin's lymphoma	Ovarian cancer (papillary serous carcinoma of borderline malignancy)	Medullary breast cancer	Breast cancer
Oocytes retrieved (n)	13	7	9	16
Freezing protocol	Slow freezing	Slow freezing	Vitrification (after transplantation of ovarian tissue)	Slow freezing
Oocytes cryopreserved (n)	12	7	1° cycle: 5 2° cycle: 4	14
Oocytes thawed (n)	1° cycle: 5 2° cycle: 4 3° cycle: 4	3	1° cycle: 5 2° cycle: 4	4
Oocytes survived (n)	1° cycle: 4 2° cycle: 2 3° cycle: 4	3	1° cycle: 5 2° cycle: 4	4
Oocytes fertilized (n)	1° cycle: 4 2° cycle: 2 3° cycle: 3	3	7	3
Embryos transferred (n)	1° cycle: 4 2° cycle: 2 3° cycle: 3	3	2	3
Clinical pregnancy (n)	1° cycle: no 2° cycle: no (biochemical pregnancy) 3° cycle: yes	Yes (twin pregnancy)	Yes (twin pregnancy)	Yes
Live birth (n)	1 (healthy male at 37 weeks' gestation)	2 (healthy females at 38 weeks' gestation)	2 (healthy boys at 33 weeks' gestation)	1 (healthy male at 37 weeks' gestation)
Mode of delivery	Spontaneous delivery	Elective Cesarean section	Elective Cesarean section	Cesarean section mild gestosis
Weight	3062 g	2100 g, 2400 g	1650 g, 1830 g	3080 g

vesicle stage, because the potential of oocyte maturation is reduced when immature oocytes are cryopreserved (Cao and Chian, 2009).

Recently, several studies have been carried out to investigate oocyte vitrification after IVM of immature oocytes. In 2007 Huang reported the successful vitrification of three in vitro matured oocytes as a strategy of fertility preservation in women with borderline ovarian malignancy (Huang *et al.*, 2007a). The first live birth after vitrification of in vitro matured oocytes is due to Chian *et al.* (2009), who achieved the birth of a healthy baby weighing 3480 g at term gestation following the recovery of 18 oocytes at the germinal vesicle stage. Sixteen out of 18 oocytes reached maturity and were vitrified; 4 oocyte survived after thawing, enabling the transfer of 3 embryos (Chian *et al.*, 2009).

Another strategy for fertility preservation is the use of immature oocytes harvested from ovarian biopsy specimens and vitrified following IVM. This technique has been applied by Huang *et al.* (2008b) in four cancer patients, achieving a mean maturation rate of 79%. In total, eight oocytes were vitrified (Huang *et al.*, 2008b).

A new approach to the freezing of immature oocytes for preventing infertility provides the ability to recover oocytes from the luteal phase of the menstrual cycle and following IVM (Demirtas *et al.*, 2008; Oktay *et al.*, 2008). The rationale for this intervention is the need to shorten the waiting time before antineoplastic treatment.

On the whole, IVM associated with cryopreservation of oocytes is a promising fertility preservation strategy for women who cannot undergo stimulation cycle for IVF, because it allows the complete avoidance of the potentially negative effects of drugs used in the ovarian stimulation and enables the freezing of oocytes within a short time period, so that the anticancer treatment can be started as soon as possible.

Despite these good assumptions and the growing number of IVM/oocyte cryopreservation cycles (the McGill Reproductive Centre has applied the technique in 70 patients with malignancies) (Ata *et al.*, 2010), we do not have actual clinical results in terms of pregnancies and live births in patients with malignancies that can be used to confirm the efficiency of the technique. Moreover, overall pregnancy rates in the other groups of patients (mainly patients at high risk of ovarian hyperstimulation syndrome [OHSS]) remain lower than those achieved in IVF cycles, suggesting the need for further development of the IVM/cryopreservation technique before it is included among the reliable options for fertility preservation.

The same technique of oocyte cryopreservation allowed the vitrification of eight oocytes to save fertility in a patient with Turner's syndrome (Huang *et al.*, 2008a), a genetic pathology that affects about 50/100 000 females' live births. Turner's syndrome is characterized by highly variable genetic anomalies that consist in a partial or complete deletion of the X sexual chromosome; it can be present as a monosomy or as a mosaicism with two or three different cellular lines. Fifty percent of Turner's syndrome patients have a 45 X0 karyotype, while the remaining cases have karyotypes with mosaicism or X isochromosome or with partial or whole Y chromosomes. Turner's syndrome is classified among the conditions of premature ovarian failure (POF). The number of germinal cells is normal until 18 weeks of gestation; then the degeneration process begins. From early childhood (2–5 years) increased levels of FSH and luteinizing hormone (LH) are detected and in the adult age these reach menopausal levels.

Up to 30% of patients with Turner's syndrome show sign of pubertal development and 2–5% present regular menstrual cycles without therapy. Two percent of these patients have a spontaneous pregnancy (Hjerrild *et al.*, 2008). Recently, some ovarian follicles have also been observed in 12- to 19-year-old females with monosomy 45 X0. Aso *et al.* (2010) investigated the possibility of predicting a spontaneous menarche and regular menstrual cycles in 50 patients with Turner's syndrome. The patients were divided into three groups: in the first group were patients with spontaneous menarche before 16 years and regular cycles for at least 18 months; in the second were patients with spontaneous menarche before 16 years but irregular cycles and secondary amenorrhea; and in the third were patients without spontaneous breast development before 14 years or with primary amenorrhea at 16 years. The authors analyzed the levels of FSH and LH in these patients at 12–13 years. The results confirmed that the patients with a karyotype with mosaicism more frequently have regular cycles. The patients with FSH levels lower than 10 mIU/ml at the age of 12 years presented with spontaneous menarche and regular menstrual cycles. These results confirm the significance of high FSH levels as a preventive factor of spontaneous menarche and regular cycles. Other factors that predict premature ovarian failure are the absence of spontaneous menarche, hypoplastic ovaries or reduced development of the uterus (Pasquino *et al.*, 1997).

The occurrence of spontaneous pubertal development is directly associated with the presence of the second X chromosome in the karyotype; in fact the patients with X monosomy have a much lower incidence of spontaneous puberty than patients with mosaicism (Pasquino *et al.*, 1997). Purushothaman *et al.* (2010) confirmed that some karyotypes, including monosomy 45 X0, Xq deletions and 46 XY mosaicism, are associated with a poor fertility potential, while other karyotypes, such as 46 XX mosaicism and terminal Xp deletions, are more frequently related to spontaneous menarche. However, in a recent study by the US National Institute of Health, spontaneous pregnancies in women with 45 X0 karyotype, the classic form of Turner's syndrome, were observed. In fact, four of the five patients with spontaneous pregnancy had a 45 X0 karyotype in 49 cells of 50 cells analyzed and presented with spontaneous menarche and normal pubertal development. The presence of spontaneous fertility in this group of patients suggests that there are different alleles involved in the regulation of the fertility, placed in different positions from the X chromosome (Hadnott *et al.*, 2011). A Swedish study describes pregnancies in 12% of women with Turner's syndrome (57/482), with a live birthrate of 54% in 124 pregnancies. Forty percent (23/57) of pregnancies were spontaneous, 5% (3/57) were obtained with IVF, 2% (1/57) were obtained with intrauterine insemination (IUI) and 53% (30/57) with oocyte donation (Bryman *et al.*, 2011).

Fertility preservation can be achieved by four different methods: oocyte donation, oocyte cryopreservation, embryo cryopreservation and heterologous transplantation of ovarian tissue. Embryo cryopreservation after ovarian stimulation is the only treatment encoded by the Ethics Committee of the ASRM to preserve fertility in patients with Turner's syndrome, but this method can not be applied in prepubertal patients. In these patients, the only possible methods are oocyte and ovarian tissue cryopreservation. The purpose of ovarian tissue cryopreservation is the recovery of primordial follicles in the ovarian cortex before the end of the atretic process in order to culture them in vitro (Abir *et al.*, 2001; Gosden, 2002). The primordial and primary follicles are liable to damage and atresia during freezing, while preovulatory antral follicles which contain immature oocytes at the germinal stage do not usually survive the ovarian tissue cryopreservation procedure (Hreinsson *et al.*, 2002). Although an elevated number of follicles can be preserved with this method, the clinical efficacy of ovarian tissue cryopreservation needs to be confirmed.

An accurate selection of Turner's syndrome patients who can be submitted to a treatment of fertility preservation is very important. The discussion about the appropriateness of performing these treatments in patients with karyotype without mosaicism is still open. Hreinsson *et al.* (2002) suggested that cryopreservation of ovarian tissue from these patients should be performed at the age of 12–13 years to obtain a relevant number of primordial follicles; 90% of the patients with X0 karyotype already had FSH levels above 40 mIU/ml in prepubertal age. The ideal age to perform the oocyte or ovarian tissue cryopreservation is not yet established, but some authors suggest that the age of 12–14 years is more suitable (El-Shawarby *et al.*, 2010). Another study (Abir *et al.*, 2001) suggests that the ovarian tissue cryopreservation should be performed even before the first signs of puberty, since most of the follicles might already be lost at the beginning of puberty. Overall the biopsy is an invasive method that should be reserved only for selected patients; at the beginning, the evaluation of ovarian reserve should be done through non-invasive methods such as plasmatic screening of FSH, AMH and inhibin B. The extent and rate of decline of the plasmatic level of AMH, the reduction of inhibin B and the increase of FSH are associated with ovarian failure. In particular, AMH which is expressed from granulosa cells of the follicles in the first maturation stage is a predictive marker of ovarian reserve; further studies are needed to establish the sensibility and specificity of this marker (Purushothaman *et al.*, 2010). A study by Hagen *et al.* (2010) showed a close association between levels of AMH and ovarian reserve. Turner's syndrome patients with X monosomy or with absence of spontaneous pubertal development and premature ovarian failure were found to have already very low levels of AMH before 25 years of age (AMH < 2–7 pmol/l). On the contrary, patients with mosaicism or with preserved ovarian function had normal levels of AMH.

Another treatment to preserve fertility in these patients is heterologous transplantation of ovarian tissue; Mhatre and Mhatre (2006) described the first case of transplantation of ovarian tissue from a mother to her 15-year-old-daughter with Turner's syndrome. The menstrual cycles returned for 12 months. Additional studies are needed to evaluate the effects of immunosuppressive therapy on ovarian function in the following years.

Lau *et al.* (2009) recently described the application of oocyte cryopreservation for patients with Turner's syndrome. In this study the reproductive state of 28 patients was analyzed; 46% of the patients had partial or complete deletion of an X chromosome, 32% had mosaicism, and 21% X isochromosome or X ring chromosome. The age of diagnosis was variable; 21% of cases were diagnosed in prenatal or neonatal age, 21% were diagnosed between 6 months and 10 years, while 57% were diagnosed between 11 and 20 years. Six patients (21%) had spontaneous pubertal development: five of these had mosaicism whereas one with monosomy X had reached the stage of development Tanner 2. Fourteen percent (all with mosaicism karyotype) had a spontaneous menarche. In 7 out of 21 patients, an ultrasound exam showed regular uterine and ovarian morphology; only one of these patients had a karyotype with X monosomy. The levels of FSH were examined in 21 patients and were associated with karyotype. Ten of eleven patients (91%) with karyotype 45 X0 had levels of FSH greater than 40 IU/ml, whereas two of four patients with X isochromosome or X ring chromosome had levels of FSH lower than 40 IU/ml. The mean plasma concentration of FSH in the group with mosaicism karyotype was found to be significantly lower than in the group with karyotype monosomy X or X ring chromosome (25.9 ± 10.4 IU/l vs. 80.7 ± 8.0 IU/l and 53.9 ± 19.2 IU/l, $P < 0.05$). There was a direct correlation between the increase in FSH levels and increasing age in the patients with karyotype 45 X0: the increase in FSH levels above 40 IU/l appeared at the age of about 16 years. Based on the criteria listed above, four patients (14%) were deemed to be suitable for fertility preservation.

One of the four selected patients (patient 4) underwent ovarian stimulation with a gonadotropin-releasing hormone (GnRH) agonist and recombinant FSH 450 IU for five days and then 600 IU for another five days. Two oocytes at the stage of metaphase II were recovered at the oocyte retrieval and were vitrified (Lau *et al.*, 2009). Moreover, El-Shawarby *et al.* (2010) treated a 22-year-old patient with mosaic Turner's syndrome and obtained eight oocytes that were vitrified for future use. These results confirm previous observations of Abir *et al.* (2001): the preservation of fertility should be suggested to patients with mosaicism or X isochromosome. However, the discussion about the patients with X monosomy is still open. Similarly, further evidence is needed to identify the appropriate age for oocyte cryopreservation.

The selection of patients whose oocytes are suitable for cryopreservation can be done through the evaluation of predictive factors for the presence of ovarian follicles, as hypothesized by Borgrstrom *et al.* (2009). Fifty-seven patients with Turner's syndrome, aged between 8 and 19.8 years, underwent laparoscopic ovarian biopsy. In 15 patients (26%) some follicles in the analyzed ovarian tissue were recovered (86% with mosaicism, 10.7% with X monosomy), whereas 8 of 13 patients (62%) with spontaneous menarche and 11 of 19 (58%) with spontaneous pubertal development had some follicles. The higher percentage of follicular presence was in the women aged between 12 and 16 years. The patients with some ovarian follicles more often had normal values of FSH and low levels of AMH.

Therefore, spontaneous pubertal development, mosaicism and normal hormone levels are significantly associated with a higher probability of having ovarian follicles; consequently, they can be used as screening factors to identify patients suitable for ovarian biopsy. Recently Huang *et al.* (2008a) proposed a combination of ovarian tissue cryopreservation and oocyte cryopreservation to preserve fertility in Turner's syndrome. They described a case of a 16-year-old patient with Turner's syndrome (karyotype 45 X [20%]/46 XX [80%]) submitted for the retrieval of 11 immature oocytes from the ovarian cortex; 8 of these oocytes were vitrified after IVM (maturation rate: 73%) (Huang *et al.*, 2008a).

The application of methods to preserve fertility in Turner's syndrome should be associated with suitable counseling about the risks of the pregnancy in these patients. In fact, pregnancy in Turner's syndrome is associated with higher risks of miscarriages, congenital malformations, hypertension and dissection of the aorta and with increased maternal death. The risk of fetal loss and congenital malformations is increased both in spontaneous pregnancies and in pregnancies obtained through oocyte donation. In a review by Tarani *et al.* (1998) that included 160 spontaneous pregnancies in patients with Turner's syndrome, the incidence of fetal loss, chromosomal abnormalities and congenital malformations and perinatal death were 29%, 20% and 7%, respectively. Birkebaek *et al.* (2002) analyzed the reproductive state of 412 women with Turner's syndrome by consulting the data of the Danish Cytogenetic Central Register. Thirty-three of these women (only one with 45 X0 karyotype, 27 with mosaicism and 5 with structural anomalies of the second X chromosome) have given birth to 64 children. The karyotype of 25 of these children was analyzed and in six cases a chromosomal anomaly was diagnosed (24%). Other studies show a higher incidence of trisomy 21 (4% vs. 0.4% in the general population) and Turner's syndrome (15% vs. 0.5% in the general population) in offspring of patients with Turner's syndrome (King *et al.*, 1978; Nielsen *et al.*, 1979; Swapp *et al.*, 1989). The increased incidence of chromosomal anomalies in these fetuses could be one of the possible causes of the increased spontaneous abortion rate observed in Turner's syndrome; other possible factors are uterine malformations, reduced uterine development, reduced uterine vascular perfusion, reduced endometrial receptivity and the presence of autoantibodies that correlate with the higher incidence of autoimmune pathologies in Turner's syndrome patients. Further studies (Khastgir *et al.*, 1997) have documented a higher incidence of miscarriages in patients with Turner's syndrome who underwent cycles of oocyte donation. This finding confirms that the major incidence of uterine anomalies in these patients represents an important cause of miscarriage. The age of the recipients who underwent cycles of oocyte donation did not seem to influence the success rates.

Bakalov *et al.* (2007) have evaluated the association between uterine development in Turner's syndrome and hormone replacement therapy (HRT). The normal uterine development observed in Turner's syndrome patients with spontaneous pubertal development would exclude the existence of an intrinsic uterine defect that previous studies have suggested (Yaron *et al.*, 1996). The uterine development in Turner's syndrome seems rather to be related to the administration of HRT, as was demonstrated in 86 women with Turner's syndrome, aged 18–45 years, who underwent ultrasound examination of the uterus. About 1/4 (24.4%) of the women had a normal uterine development while most (44.2%) had a small uterus and 1/3 (31.4%) had an immature uterus. The patients that took HRT had a significantly larger uterus than the patients who used oral contraception or who did not receive therapy. Duration and typology of HRT influenced the uterine development; the treatments that included estradiol showed the highest efficacy.

The age of first exposure to estrogens, the stature and weight of the patient and the previous intake of growth hormone do not seem to be related to uterine measures, but previous studies recommended initiation of estrogen therapy at the age of 12–15 years. Karyotype did not show association with uterine dimensions, in contrast to suggestions from previous studies (Doerr *et al.*, 2005; Bakalov *et al.*, 2007) that showed a correlation between normal uterine development and mosaicism.

The available data about pregnancies in Turner's syndrome patients are still limited. A retrospective study of Bodri *et al.* (2006) analyzed the outcomes of pregnancies in 21 patients with Turner's syndrome who underwent 30 cycles of oocyte donation between 2001 and 2004. Among the 17 pregnancies obtained, 12 were clinical, with a high rate of biochemical miscarriage (29% vs. 12.9% in the general population). The implantation and pregnancy rate were 22% (15 of 68) and 30% (9 of 30), respectively. Premature birthrate was 50% and intrauterine growth retardation was found in 55.5% of fetuses. Hypertension was diagnosed in five of eight pregnancies and there were three cases of preeclampsia. The increased incidence of hypertensive disease in this group of patients, which was also observed in previous studies (Foudila *et al.*, 1999; Bodri *et al.*, 2006), is not related to increased maternal age or high incidence of multiple pregnancies, as is the case in the general population who undergo oocyte donation. All the patients underwent Cesarean section because of preeclampsia (two cases) and fetopelvic disproportion (the remaining). Fetopelvic disproportion has been described as the main indication for Cesarean section in different studies (Oktay *et al.*, 2010; Hadnott *et al.*, 2011).

These data suggest that pregnancies achieved in patients with Turner's syndrome require careful monitoring and that multiple pregnancies, which are associated with an increased rate of hypertensive disease, should be avoided. The risk of maternal death in a pregnancy obtained through oocyte donation is about 2%; seven cases of aortic dissection during the pregnancy were reported in the literature. The hyperdynamic and hypervolemic vascular states associated with the pregnancy seem to increase the risk of dissection of the aorta. Moreover, the gravidical hyperestrogenism can change the structural integrity of the aorta and make it more susceptible to damage. The risk of aortic dissection is increased in the early weeks of the pregnancy and in the third trimester. Boissonnas *et al.* (2009) reported a case of a patient with Turner's syndrome (45 X0–46 XY karyotype) who had achieved a pregnancy from oocyte donation. The patient underwent a cardiac screening before the pregnancy which returned a normal result, but had dissection of the aorta at 38 weeks of gestation after the diagnosis of bicuspid aortic valve at 16 weeks of gestation.

The ASRM recommends cardiac screening in all patients with Turner's syndrome who want to become pregnant. The screening should include echocardiography, ECG and magnetic resonance. The detection of a severe cardiac anomaly should represent a contra-indication to assisted reproduction in this group of patients. In patients with Turner's syndrome that undergo ART, single embryo transfer should be performed in order to avoid the hemodynamic overload associated with multiple pregnancies (Bondy, 2007). Recently the FCOG (French College of Obstetricians and Gynaecologists) formed a committee that included the French Societies of Obstetrics and Gynaecology, Cardiology, Cardiac Surgery and Vascular Surgery, Anesthesia, Endocrinology, the Study Group on Oocyte Donation and the Biochemical Agency, with the aim to establish guidelines about the management of patients with Turner's syndrome before and during the pregnancy. The recommendations include a list of the exams required before the pregnancy, the information for the patients, the indications about monitoring of the pregnancy and type of delivery, as well as postnatal follow-up (Cabanes *et al.*, 2010).

IVF laboratory flexibility indication

Unexpected events may often occur during the daily operations of an assisted reproduction center which prevent routine insemination of the oocytes recovered. There may, for instance, be a lack of seminal fluid (sperm). Another possibility could be the failure to recover sperm from a surgical procedure. In these cases, temporary oocyte freezing salvages the treatment cycle. Furthermore, frozen oocytes and sperm make extracorporeal fertilization possible without the presence of the patients. In addition, if a cycle of intrauterine insemination has to be cancelled as a result of excessive follicular development with the risk of a multiple pregnancy, the cycle may be saved by harvesting and freezing the oocytes.

Oocyte cryopreservation allows more flexibility in the daily operations of assisted reproduction procedures. The success of this option was first documented more than 10 years ago when pregnancies from frozen oocytes and epididymal, testicular or frozen sperms were reported (Porcu *et al.*, 1999a, 1999b, 2000a).

The controversial family planning indication

In modern societies the proportion of women who delay childbearing beyond the age of 35 years has greatly increased in recent decades (UK Office for National Statistics, 2008). The impressive recent rise in the mean maternal age is the result of postponing the first birth rather than a rise in fertility at later ages. Similar changes can be observed in most developed countries and thus, in Canada, most women will deliver their first child over the age of 30 with the proportions of first births after age 34 increasing from 6% (1975) to 18% (1995) to 25% in 2005 (Leader, 2006). Also, in the United States the number of first births per 1000 women aged 35–39 increased by 36% between 1991 and 2001, and the rate among women aged 40–44 leapt by a remarkable 70% (Balash and Gratacós, 2011). The occidental society, career aspirations and opportunities, and the difficulties in achieving economic stability are just some of the factors responsible for the increase in mean maternal age in the search of pregnancy.

Unfortunately the female reproductive system is particularly sensitive to the toll of time; a quantitative decline in oocyte reserves and a qualitative deterioration in the residual eggs together have been identified as the salient processes that underlie reproductive compromise in aging women (Doherty and Pal, 2011). Pregnancy rate, in fact, decreases exponentially after maternal age of 37 years and the decline is accelerated after 40 years; this age-related decline is probably associated with the poorer oocyte quality (Committee on Gynecologic Practice of American College of Obstetricians and Gynecologists, 2008). It has been hypothesized that there is a fixed window of 13 years before menopause, during which accelerated ovarian atresia takes place. Accordingly, women who are destined to go through menopause at the age of 45 years (10% of the population) might be expected to have accelerated atresia and reduced fecundity beginning at the age of 32 years (Nikolaou and Templeton, 2003). The relationship between pregnancy rates and oocyte quality is confirmed by the pregnancy rates registered in cycles of oocyte donation, which are strictly correlated with the donor age.

Women often tend to think that advances in new reproductive technologies can compensate for the age-related decline in fertility and are not aware that age remains the single most important determinant of male and female fertility, either natural or treated. The influence of age on fertility is particularly severe in women, but also applies to men, who have a constant decline in fertility starting from the age of 39, with a reduction of 21–23% every year (Matorras *et al.*, 2011). Oocyte cryopreservation allows a woman to freeze her own younger and healthier eggs for the future, preserving her fertility and giving her the opportunity to postpone pregnancy. The medical indications for oocyte cryopreservation are all the conditions at high risk of premature ovarian failure, such as antineoplastic treatments, genetic diseases (Turner's syndrome), endometriosis and ovarian surgery and idiopathic premature ovarian failure.

Changes in demographics, the role of women in society, career aspirations and economic upheavals are all recognized as contributory factors to the global trend to "postpone pregnancy," which represents a social indication for oocyte cryopreservation.

The cryopreservation of oocytes at a young age could allow women not only to achieve a higher education and a better career for personal fulfillment, but also to contribute to family earnings in order to achieve economic stability before having a child. In addition to this, a lot of women delay a pregnancy because they encounter difficulties in finding the "right partner" in young age. On the whole, egg freezing could have many benefits for women who want to postpone pregnancy:

- It allows them to plan their professional life with calmness and serenity
- It allows them to have a child when there is economic stability
- It is associated with a reduction in the incidence of chromosomal abnormalities which is strictly related with the age of the oocytes.

At the same time, oocyte cryopreservation for social reasons raises some problems because it is a medical and surgical treatment that is applied to healthy women and can be associated with some complications such as OHSS or bleeding. Moreover, pregnancy in women aged over 40 years is complicated by a higher risk of preeclampsia, chronic hypertension, cardiac disease and perinatal complications (Goold and Savulescu, 2009; Balash and Gratacós, 2011).

The first reported study about women's motivation for egg freezing showed that 50% felt pressured by their biological clock and 15% considered egg freezing as an insurance policy (Goold and Savulescu, 2009). Another survey showed the attitude of 1914 women aged between 21 and 40 years toward egg freezing; 31.5% of women interviewed considered themselves as potential social oocyte freezers, whereas 3.1% would definitely consider the procedure (Stoop *et al.*, 2011).

Different objections have been raised against oocyte cryopreservation for social reasons. First of all, older women are more likely to die while the child is still quite young, leaving him/her an orphan; moreover, children of older parents will have to face the burden of caring for their parents at an earlier stage of their lives than children of younger parents. To date, the public health message in relation to deferring childbearing should be to inform patients of the risks associated with a pregnancy in advanced age, educate women about reproduction and cautiously encourage conception at a younger age. It is particularly important to explain to the patients in a clear manner the implications of oocyte cryopreservation and the potential failure of the technique, in order to avoid unrealistic expectations and unjustified delays of reproduction.

Chapter 2

The evolution of human oocyte cryopreservation

Preliminary research

Since the first successful human embryo cryopreservation 25 years ago, it has often been underlined that freezing of excess embryos is only a temporary solution with many disadvantages and that it would often be more acceptable to store human oocytes to avoid ethical and legal problems. Indeed, shortly after the first birth with frozen human embryos, the same clinical success with frozen human oocytes was announced. However, the enthusiasm for the announcement of the first pregnancies with frozen eggs was not followed by a rapid incorporation of the technique into the in vitro fertilization (IVF) clinical routine and, unlike the early and fast spreading of embryo freezing, oocyte cryopreservation was, and still is, considered as an experimental technique. Lessons from the general history of IVF have taught us that techniques truly indispensable for solving a problem have been rapidly adopted in the clinical routine before evidence of their safety has been confirmed. Embryo cryopreservation was developed because of the unavoidable choice "freezing or wasting." On the contrary, oocyte cryopreservation was an optional choice. Ethical concerns were not powerful enough to push clinical research and application in oocyte cryopreservation. This is the main reason why those early, fully successful clinical applications remained anecdotal. The postulated intrinsic cryovulnerability of the mature oocyte raised safety concerns which became a major restraint. It was thanks to the basic biological studies of excellent researchers in reproductive cryobiology that many of those concerns were alleviated in the 1990s, allowing the clinical resumption of oocyte cryopreservation by the end of that decade. A relatively intensive and, in some cases, routine application only has been performed in Italy, due to the recent restrictive legal regulation of IVF in that country. Variations in the results reported from different countries and teams make it still difficult to measure the true success of the procedure even though, in some reports, oocyte cryopreservation seems to equal embryo freezing in efficiency. In the past few years, the clinical application of egg storage was partially shifted to vitrification, despite the absence of sufficient basic biological studies addressing safety issues. Recently, the proposal of novel applications, such as the debated egg storage for non-medical indications to postpone maternity in young women, as well as the development of commercial interests, prompted acceleration in the rise in oocyte cryopreservation.

Early animal studies

Studies concerning the cryopreservation of oocytes and the effects of low temperatures on cell biology have been undertaken since the end of the 1940s, yielding knowledge that have had a practical as well as theoretical significance. Chang (1948a, 1948b) documented the ability of rabbit oocytes stored at either 10 °C or 0 °C to generate embryos and healthy offspring. Since then, however, the author has observed that pregnancy occurred more frequently with embryos kept at low temperature (11–37% after 24 hours' storage) than with eggs (3–11% after storage for 6–31 hours). Subsequently, Chang (1953) published further investigations on egg storage at low temperature. Rabbit eggs were taken from the tubes of albino rabbits and placed in a suspension containing an equivalent percentage of "Ringer" solution and rabbit serum. Some of the oocytes (130) were kept in test tubes for 30–31 hours at a temperature of $10\,°C$, while the remaining 137 oocytes were kept at $0\,°C$, after an initial acclimatization time of one hour at $10\,°C$. Oocytes stored at $10\,°C$ were transferred to the left tuba and oocytes stored at $0\,°C$ to the right tuba. No statistically significant difference was seen between the effects of conservation at $0\,°C$ or $10\,°C$. Both groups registered a low rate of normal fertilization, 7% of transferred oocytes in the first group and 4% in the second group, after 31 hours of preservation. This was statistically lower than that of a control group (27%). These observations raised the possibility of damage resulting from cell storage at low temperatures.

Sherman and Lin (1958) evaluated the effect of glycerol supplementation on low temperature preservation of mouse eggs. They observed that some germ cells can survive exposure to a temperature of $-10\,°C$ if 5% glycerol is added to the storage solution consisting of 500 ml of distilled water, 3.38 g of sodium chloride, 0.09 g of calcium chloride, 0.16 g of potassium chloride, 0.05 g sodium bicarbonate and 0.36 g dextrose (modified Locke solution). The glycerol lowers the freezing point preventing the medium from freezing. One hundred and eighty oocytes were transferred into 30 mice recipients, with 17% embryo development after one hour of storage and 5% after two hours. The same study analyzed the effects of glycerol's presence inside the cell on the ability of oocytes to generate offspring after transfer to receiving mice. The penetration of glycerol into the cells was achieved through exposure to a 5% glycerol solution for 15 minutes. Exposure to glycerol solution first caused oocyte shrinkage followed by recovery to their initial volume after 8–10 minutes. Sixty oocytes were transferred into 10 mice recipients and 6 pregnancies were achieved. Therefore, the presence of glycerol inside the cells did not jeopardize fertilization and embryo development.

In another study, Sherman (1959) carried out an assessment of the survival and function of mouse egg cells after a rapid reduction in temperature and storage at low temperatures. Altogether 1858 oocytes, harvested from the tubes of brown female mice, after hyperstimulation, were transferred into 310 white mice recipients. Prior to transfer the egg cells of the study group were released into the storage medium; some were cooled to $0\,°C$ at a rate of $0.2\,°C$ per second and the remainder to a temperature of $-21\,°C$ at a speed of $1\,°C$ per second. The cells were then restored to a temperature of $22\,°C$ and transferred to recipients. In the control group cells were preserved at a temperature of $22\,°C$. The rate of pregnancy and survival of egg cells, along with their reproductive capacity, were unaffected by the rapid lowering of temperature.

However, egg cells proved extremely sensitive to prolonged exposure to low temperatures: with increasing exposure time, the rate of survival dramatically decreased.

Shortly after, Burks (1965) reported on the morphology of cryopreserved human and rabbit egg cells subjected to freezing. Four hundred and fifty-five rabbit eggs were divided into groups and subjected to increasing concentrations of glycerol (0%, 10%, and 35%) in Locke's solution at different temperatures ($5\,°C$, $22\,°C$, and $37\,°C$, for 15 minutes). The cells were then stored in sealed glass containers and immersed in liquid nitrogen. Morphological evaluation was performed after 1–15 days of storage. The survival cytological criteria were: (1) integrity of the vitelline membrane and the zona pellucida, (2) absence of granulation and/or deformation of the cytoplasm. The highest survival rate (96%) was recorded in egg cells exposed to 35% glycerol at a temperature of 5 °C.

In the early 1960s, Mazur (1963) conducted various studies on the kinetics of cellular dehydration in relation to changes in temperature. He worked out a differential equation relating cooling rate, surface and cell volume, membrane permeability to water and the temperature coefficient of the permeability constant. Through this equation it is possible to derive the intracellular water content and predict the probability of intracellular ice forming. The equation allows a number of conclusions:

- Larger cells with a lower surface:volume ratio have a slower dehydration speed than smaller cells because they retain more water and are more likely to encounter ice formation
- A fast rate of cooling does not allow enough water leakage from the cell, and makes intracellular crystal formation more likely
- A cell characterized by high permeability to water achieves faster dehydration.

The fate of intracellular water as the temperature changes in egg cells was evaluated in a study by Asahina (1961), which showed that the intracellular content of the sea urchin egg cell did not start to freeze until it reached a temperature of −5 °C; if cooling continued at a rate of 1 °C/min, cells did not freeze but suffered a gradual decline in volume, while increasing the cooling rate to 10 °C/min caused freezing and blocked the escape of water. In keeping with the Mazur equation, the trend to form intracellular crystals seems much more related to rapid changes in temperature.

In later studies, however, Mazur (1970, 1984, 1988) pointed out that inhibition of intracellular ice formation is necessary but not sufficient for the survival of the cell. Slow freezing can be injurious in itself. As ice develops outside the cells, the residual unfrozen medium forms channels of decreasing size and increasing solute concentration. The cells lie in the channels and shrink due to the osmotic response to the rising solute concentration. Previous theories ascribed slow freezing injury to the concentration of solutes and/or cell shrinkage. Recent experiments, however, indicate that the damage is due more to a decrease in the size of the unfrozen channels. In addition, the rate of warming can have as much effect on survival as the cooling rate.

The first birth from animal oocytes cryopreserved in liquid nitrogen was announced by Parkening et al. (1976) who obtained three normal mouse offspring. Whittingham (1977), too, achieved successful cryopreservation of unfertilized mouse oocytes resulting in off-spring. Hamster egg cryopreservation was also investigated. Choung (1986) evaluated the viability and fertilizability of unfertilized hamster oocytes in different freezing conditions: in the first group oocytes were placed in medium at room temperature, while the second group were placed in medium at 0 °C. They were cooled to −6 °C at a rate of −2 °C/min (method 1) or at −0.5 °C/min (method 2). After thawing, 52% (method 1) and 64% (method 2) of the oocytes showed normal morphological features. The fertilization rate of frozen-thawed oocytes was 26%, while the penetration rate proved to be one-third that of fresh oocytes. Critser (1986) conducted three experiments to evaluate the effects of vitrification (Rall and Fahy, 1985) or slow freezing on human sperm penetration of zona-free hamster oocytes. The survival of hamster oocytes, as defined by observation of morphological features, did not differ between the vitrification and the freezing groups. However, vitrified oocytes showed a lower frequency of sperm penetration than frozen oocytes (Critser, 1986).

Early human studies

Burks (1965), encouraged by his good results with rabbit oocyte cryopreservation, performed a subsequent experiment with human oocytes. Ten human eggs were exposed to 35% glycerol at a temperature of 5 °C and then frozen in liquid nitrogen. After thawing, 9 out of 10 eggs survived (90%).

Trounson (1986) examined different methods of human oocyte cryopreservation. Part of the experiment was carried out with aged oocytes which had failed to become fertilized in the routine IVF program. Slow cooling with 1.5 M dimethyl sulfoxide (DMSO) gave 18% survival. Rapid cooling with 1.5 M DMSO gave 25% survival. Ultrarapid cooling with 1.5 M DMSO and 3.0 M resulted in 52% egg survival. Vitrification gave rise to a 75% survival rate. The second part of the experiment was performed with mature human oocytes. No survival was registered after slow cooling with 1.5 M DMSO. Slow cooling with 1.5 M 1,2-propanediol (PROH) gave good results with 67% survival and 100% fertilization. Vitrification after removing cumulus cells resulted in a 67% survival rate and 75% fertilization rate without subsequent cleavage. Vitrification with the cumulus intact was followed by fertilization and embryo development to at least the eight-cell stage. Therefore, even though small numbers of mature oocytes were involved in these experiments, it has been shown that human oocytes may survive freezing and thawing and be fertilized after insemination. Furthermore, those early experiments gave indications about the most efficient methods of human egg cryopreservation. Unfortunately, despite the development of these methods for egg cryopreservation in mid 1985, Trounson's group has been unable to transfer developing embryos to patients because of legal restrictions in the Victorian State.

Chen (1986) reported the first human pregnancy with cryopreserved oocytes. In his oocyte cryopreservation program, Chen adopted a slow freezing/rapid thawing protocol with DMSO as a cryoprotectant. After the reduction in size of the oocyte/cumulus oophorus complex, 1.5 M DMSO was added as a one-step procedure. Seeding was performed at −7 °C followed by slow cooling between −7 °C and −36 °C, rapid freezing to −196 °C and storage in liquid nitrogen. Rapid thawing in a 37 °C water-bath was followed by dilution of the DMSO as a single step by adding four times the sample volume of phosphate-buffered saline. The oocyte was examined for morphological evidence of survival. The further development of the oocyte required the transfer to the regular culture medium, and at the appropriate time insemination was carried out.

Thirty-eight out of fifty (76%) cryopreserved oocytes survived thawing, 71% were fertilized and 85% cleaved even to 6–8 cells (Chen, 1988). Transfers of between two and three embryos derived from frozen-thawed oocytes were performed in seven patients and two pregnancies (one twin and one single) resulted. With regards to the first patient who became pregnant, a 29-year-old woman, six eggs were frozen, three were thawed, survived and were fertilized. Three embryos were transferred at the three-cell to four-cell stages, about 46 hours after insemination. A twin pregnancy was achieved with the birth of two healthy children. The second patient, aged 37 years, conceived with the same technique using her spare eggs, which had been kept frozen for four months. She delivered a healthy female. Therefore, Chen's clinical results led to a pregnancy rate of 29% embryo transfers and a birthrate of 6% thawed oocytes.

Al-Hasani et al. (1986) cryopreserved 133 oocytes of varying quality from 22 patients. The survival rate achieved after thawing was 34%, while the in vitro fertilization rate was 75%.

Out of a total of seven embryo transfers there was one pregnancy following the replacement of a six-cell embryo.

Van Uem *et al.* (1987) published the second birth reported in the literature after oocyte cryopreservation with an alternative freezing technique. In an attempt to overcome cell damage due to supercooling, he developed a computer-controlled "open-vessel" freezing device (CTE 8100). This device, using tailed plastic straws, permits seeding to take place automatically in the ideal temperature range around the freezing point of the medium ("self-seeding"). Further, van Uem adopted the technique of slow freezing and slow thawing. As Chen did, van Uem also reduced the cumulus by needle dissection. A freezing medium of phosphate-buffered saline containing 10% heat-inactivated fetal cord serum and 1.5 M DMSO not chilled before the addition to the oocyte was used. Seven out of twenty-eight (25%) frozen oocytes survived after thawing.

A further study of Al-Hasani *et al.* (1987) describes the results of three freezing methods used for cryopreserving 320 human oocytes. The first method was a slow freezing protocol and used 1.5 M DMSO and 20% inactivated fetal calf serum. In the second method of slow freezing, the cryoprotectant was 1.5 M PROH and 0.1 M sucrose. The third method with ultrarapid freezing used 3 M DMSO plus and 0.25 M sucrose. The survival and fertilization rates of the first method were 28% and 50%, respectively, with 20% polyploidy. The survival and fertilization rates of the second method were 32% and 75%, respectively, with 40% polyploidy. The ultracooling method gave poor results with a survival rate of 4%.

Diedrich *et al.* (1988) published a study where 283 excess oocytes from 48 patients were frozen. After thawing, 136 out of 157 oocytes survived (87% survival rate). The viability rate of oocytes after the procedure, evaluated through morphological criteria, was 32% (43 oocytes out of 136) and the fertilization rate was 58%. Embryo transfer was performed in 11 patients, initiating two pregnancies, though both ended in abortion.

As a matter of fact, over the course of a few years during the 1980s, the knowledge about human oocyte cryopreservation had progressed greatly. The feasibility of human egg freezing was clearly demonstrated, provided the oocytes were mature and of good quality. Oocytes could undergo freezing and thawing by both slow freezing and vitrification with high survival and fertilization rates. Embryos generated from thawed oocytes could develop and implant normally and healthy children could be delivered. It is surprising and disconcerting that, despite the favorable results obtained in both basic research and clinical application, no pregnancies and births were achieved in the eight years following those early successes.

Subsequent research

At the time, the possibility of increased aneuploidy as a result of exposing mature eggs to cryoprotectants and to freezing and thawing was a concern. Depolymerization of the spindle microtubules by cryoprotectants or by cooling may prevent the normal separation of sister chromatids and fertilization, and thus lead to chromatid non-disjunction and the state of aneuploidy after the extrusion of the second polar body. Magistrini and Szollosi (1980) and Pickering and Johnson (1987) described depolymerization of the spindle microtubules induced by cooling in mouse eggs and even by transient cooling to room temperature in human oocytes (Pickering *et al.*, 1990). However, the same authors observed that the depolymerization was reversible. Vincent *et al.* (1989) found that the addition of cryoprotectant was responsible for the depolymerization of the microtubules but these changes were reversible after the removal of cryoprotectant and a short period of culture. Glenister *et al.* (1987) found that using oocytes frozen by slow cooling in DMSO did not significantly increase the incidence of aneuploid zygotes in the mouse. These data contradict the findings of Kola *et al.* (1988) who found a two- to threefold increase in aneuploidy after slow cooling in DMSO and after vitrification. Sathananthan *et al.* (1988) suggested a cautious approach to the integration of egg freezing in clinical IVF because of the sensitivity of the meiotic spindle to simple cooling, even at $0\,°C$, leading to extensive depolymerization of the microtubules. However, widespread displacement of chromosomes was not apparent in that study. These authors affirm that the results of the literature taken together clearly indicate that not all embryos or fetuses derived from frozen oocytes are abnormal. It is possible that depolymerization and repolymerization may occur in some oocytes in a way to least disturb the normal distribution and behavior of chromosomes that are suspended on the spindle during freezing and thawing.

The consensus arising from all these studies appears to be that inappropriate exposure to cryoprotectants and cooling may induce anomalies in the spindle microtubules (Aigner *et al.*, 1992; Joly *et al.*, 1992; Bernard and Fuller, 1996; Boiso *et al.*, 2002).

Because of the concern that had been raised over mature oocyte cryopreservation, some teams addressed their research towards freezing immature oocytes at the germinal vesicle stage as it was thought these oocytes would be less sensitive to cryoinjury (Mandelbaum *et al.*, 1988a; Toth *et al.*, 1994; Baka *et al.*, 1995; Son *et al.*, 1996; Park *et al.*, 1997). In actual fact, the literature did not show any true advantage of immature oocyte freezing as regards survival and fertilization rates as well as embryo developmental capacity.

In the 1990s, in parallel, the effects of cryopreservation on mature human eggs were reappraised. Several authors agreed on the fact that appropriate protocols allow the cryopreservation of mature oocytes without any significant change in the meiotic spindle and without any increase in the rate of aneuploid embryos (Gook *et al.*, 1993, 1994; Van Blerkom and Davis, 1994; George *et al.*, 1996; Cobo *et al.*, 2001). These reassuring fundamental studies should have opened the way to new clinical trials. In reality, additional doubts about possible injury to the zona pellucida (Dumoulin *et al.*, 1994; Kazem *et al.*, 1995) and cortical granules (Al-Hasani *et al.*, 1987; Vincent *et al.*, 1989; Al-Hasani and Diedrich, 1995) leading to alterations in the mechanism of fertilization and increased incidence of polyspermia were of concern.

A turning point in the efficiency of human oocyte cryopreservation was reached with the introduction of intracytoplasmic sperm injection (ICSI). Gook *et al.* (1995b) compared traditional IVF and ICSI for thawed oocyte insemination. Although no differences were seen in the percentage of normal fertilization, ICSI was found to be associated with a significantly higher cleavage rate (Gook *et al.*, 1995b). A similar study was done by Kazem *et al.* (1995) who achieved 45.9% fertilization in the ICSI group and 13.5% in the IVF group; in the IVF group, only one fertilized oocyte cleaved while in the ICSI group all the fertilized eggs cleaved.

Recent clinical application

In spite of the great increase in basic knowledge, the clinical application of oocyte cryopreservation was kept in stagnation for a long time. Unlike other techniques such as embryo cryopreservation or ICSI, which were quickly incorporated in to the clinical routine before displaying evidence of safety, oocyte cryopreservation was still regarded as an experimental procedure, potentially dangerous and unsafe. As a matter of fact, there was no urgent need for implementation of oocyte freezing in current assisted reproductive technology (ART) as embryo freezing was a reliable alternative. Similarly, ethical indications were not powerful enough to urge clinical research in oocyte cryopreservation.

It was only in the second half of the 1990s that further clinical studies were undertaken. Tucker *et al.* (1996) cryopreserved 285 aged, unfertilized oocytes with slow freezing using 1.5 M PROH and 0.1 M sucrose. Fifty-five percent of the oocytes survived thawing and were inseminated with ICSI, with a 41% fertilization rate being achieved. In the second part of the study, seven couples from their donor oocyte program consented to receive cryopreserved donated oocytes in eight thaw cycles. Cryosurvival of the 81 fresh donated oocytes was relatively poor (24.7%) but normal fertilization after ICSI was 65% and embryo development was 100%. Uterine transfer of 13 embryos in five cycles gave rise to three early pregnancies (60%), but none went successfully to term. In the following years, a number of first-ever achievements changed the clinical background of oocyte cryopreservation. Among the giants in reproductive cryobiology, Gook *et al.*'s studies (1993, 1994, 1995a, 1995b) were especially useful in alleviating concerns about the safety of oocyte cryopreservation.

The first live birth of a healthy female conceived from oocytes cryopreserved with 1.5 M PROH + sucrose 0.2 M and inseminated with ICSI was published by Porcu *et al.* (1997) at the University of Bologna. The announcement of this live birth, nearly a decade after the first reports of births following cryopreservation of human oocytes (Chen, 1986; Van Uem *et al.* 1987) reawakened interest in this field. In the following year, several reports announced pregnancies and births from oocytes cryopreserved with PROH and inseminated with ICSI (Nawroth and Kissing, 1998; Polak de Fried *et al.*, 1998; Young *et al.*, 1998). In the same year, Tucker *et al.* (1998a) published the first birth from immature cryopreserved oocytes. In this study Tucker collected and cryopreserved 29 oocytes after ovarian stimulation in a 28-year-old woman; none of the 16 mature oocytes survived thawing, while 3 of 13 germinal vesicles survived. Two out of the three oocytes reached full maturity in culture and were normal following fertilization by ICSI. A single pregnancy was achieved after transferring both embryos. An uneventful full-term gestation ended with the birth of a healthy female weighing 3300 g. Shortly afterwards, Kuleshova *et al.* (1999) published the first birth, of a healthy female, from oocytes cryopreserved with vitrification.

From then on, two main lines of clinical research were followed: slow freezing and vitrification. Initially, slow freezing was the most popular. Since 1997, ICSI had been invariably used to inseminate cryopreserved oocytes and has proven to be a suitable means of optimizing fertilization after thawing and subsequent embryo development. This was probably the key to success that opened a new era in the clinical application of oocyte cryopreservation.

Porcu's team at the University of Bologna thought it was the right time for undertaking an intensive investigation and documentation of the actual degree of clinical efficiency of using frozen eggs in humans. In the first trial, 1769 supernumerary oocytes were frozen using slow freezing with 1.5 M PROH and 0.2 M sucrose; 1502 oocytes were thawed. The overall survival rate was 54%, the fertilization rate after ICSI was 58% and the cleavage rate 91%. In a portion of the thawed oocytes, the effects of duration of cryopreservation were evaluated: no difference was seen in the survival rate following 24 hours and three months of storage (59% and 60%, respectively). Sixteen pregnancies were achieved in 112 thawing cycles. Seven singleton and two twin pregnancies ended with the birth of 11 healthy children (Porcu *et al.*,

2000a). In that early trial, it was also documented that elective cryopreservation of all the oocytes retrieved might be a valid strategy to avoid severe ovarian hyperstimulation syndrome (OHSS). A total of 384 oocytes from 20 patients at risk of OHSS were frozen. In the subsequent postponed ICSI cycles with thawed oocytes the pregnancy rate was 17.8%.

With the revived interest of those years between the 1990s and the next decade, several case reports and small series were published. Common procedures adopted in those studies were slow freezing using 1.5 M PROH and sucrose, and ICSI to inseminate the thawed eggs. Within this basic protocol, some lines of research investigated the role of different concentrations of sucrose and the role of sodium-depleted media in an attempt to improve oocyte survival and competence. Porcu's team discovered that 0.3 M sucrose seemed to improve egg survival when compared with 0.1 M and 0.2 M sucrose (Fabbri et al., 2001). With PROH + 0.1 M sucrose, pregnancies and births were reported (Nawroth and Kissing, 1998; Young et al., 1998; Wurfel et al., 1999; Chia et al., 2000; Huttelova et al., 2003; Notrica et al., 2003; Allan, 2004; Miller et al., 2004; De Geyter et al., 2007). Freezing protocols with 0.2 M sucrose were used by several authors (Porcu et al., 1997, 1999a, 1999b, 2000a; Yang et al., 1998; Winslow et al., 2001; Yang et al., 2002; Borini et al., 2004, 2006b; Levi Setti et al., 2006; Montag et al., 2006; Bianchi et al., 2007; Gook et al., 2007a) as were those with 0.3 M sucrose (Chen et al., 2002, 2005; Fosas et al., 2003; Li et al., 2005; Tjer et al., 2005; Borini et al., 2006b; Chamayou et al., 2006; De Santis et al., 2006; La Sala et al., 2006; Levi Setti et al., 2006; Barritt et al., 2007; Konc et al., 2007). As mentioned previously, in general 0.3 M sucrose seems to improve egg survival. However, differential sucrose concentrations during dehydration (0.2 M) and rehydration (0.3 M) seem to increase the implantation rate of frozen oocytes (Bianchi et al., 2007). Another modification of the cryopreservation technique involves the replacement of sodium with choline in the freezing medium. Quintans et al. (2002) used this freezing protocol and obtained a 63% survival rate, 59% fertilization rate and 25% implantation rate. They achieved six pregnancies, with the birth of two babies. Boldt et al. (2003, 2006) reported oocyte cryopreservation outcomes after the use of a sodium-depleted protocol: survival rate was 60.4%, fertilization rate was 62% and pregnancy rate was 32.4% per embryo transfer.

Until recently, it was impossible to calculate the actual efficiency of oocyte freezing because only a small number of cases were carried out and sporadic pregnancies were obtained. Variables to be taken into consideration are egg survival, fertilization, cleavage and implantation. Survival rates reported in the early literature vary widely from 25% to more than 80%, probably because a generally small number of frozen eggs were evaluated in most studies and several different procedures were used (Al-Hasani et al., 1987; Van Uem et al., 1987; Chen, 1988; Gook et al., 1993, 1994, 1995b; Kazem et al., 1995; Tucker et al., 1996). Recently, percentages of post-thaw egg viability have been relatively more consistent. Chen et al. (2004) demonstrated a significantly higher metaphase II oocyte survival when using sucrose 0.2 M compared with 0.1 M (78.3% vs. 48.9%). One of the most active groups working in oocyte cryopreservation is that led by Borini (Borini et al., 2004, 2006a, 2006b, 2007a, 2007b). This team showed 37% egg survival with 0.1 M (Borini et al., 2004) and 74.1% with 0.3 M sucrose concentration (Borini et al., 2006a). The good results with 0.3 M sucrose solution are confirmed by Fosas et al. (2003) with 89.8% survival, by Chen et al. (2005) who achieved 75% post-thaw egg viability, and by Levi Setti et al. (2006) reporting 69.9% post-thaw intact oocytes. However, the concern expressed by Paynter et al. (2005) about the possible injury derived by extreme cell shrinkage occurring in 0.3 M sucrose solution must be kept in mind.

In general, the rate of success of oocyte cryopreservation remains difficult to calculate considering the variability among different studies, but it depends more on the number of oocytes and thawing cycles and type of patient population than on the freezing protocols.

The number of births from frozen eggs increased progressively after the first case reports. Among others, the largest series should be cited. Porcu *et al.* (2000b) reported the birth of 13 healthy children. Winslow *et al.* (2001) announced the birth of 16 children after thawing 324 egg cells, which resulted in a survival rate of 68.5%, a fertilization rate of 81% and a pregnancy rate of 26.2% per transfer. Yang *et al.* (2002) obtained the birth of 14 children after thawing 158 oocytes from donor cycles, with a 71% survival rate and a pregnancy rate per transfer of 45.8%. Fosas *et al.* (2003) announced the birth of five children. In 2004 Borini *et al.* (2004) documented the birth of 13 children and in subsequent years published the birth of 4 additional children (2006b) and then of 105 babies (2007b). Porcu (2005) reported the birth of 70 children from 2750 frozen eggs, with a survival rate after thawing of 69.6%, a fertilization rate of 74%, and a pregnancy rate per transfer of 17%. Levi Setti *et al.* (2006) reported the birth of 13 children and La Sala *et al.* (2006) achieved the birth of 7 children. Finally, Konc *et al.* (2007) described the birth of three children in Hungary, with a survival rate and a fertilization rate of 80% and 81%, respectively.

Oocyte cryopreservation proved to increase the flexibility of ART procedures, allowing the use of epididymal and testicular sperm (Porcu *et al.*, 1999a, 1999b), the use of both frozen male and female gametes (Porcu *et al.*, 2000a) and the possibility of refreezing zygotes and embryos derived from cryopreserved eggs and sperm (Azambuja *et al.*, 2005; Levi Setti *et al.* 2005; Tjer *et al.*, 2005; Montag *et al.*, 2006; Gook *et al.* 2007a).

Oocyte cryopreservation also proved to be a suitable choice for fertility preservation in oncological patients. Porcu *et al.* (2004) documented the collection and storage of an average of 15 oocytes from young oncological patients undergoing chemotherapy. The reports of the first births demonstrate that oocyte cryopreservation in oncology is a reliable option. Yang *et al.* (2007) documented the first birth in a gestational carrier who conceived with frozen oocytes belonging to a patient with Hodgkin's lymphoma. This patient under-went egg retrieval before radiotherapy and the eggs were cryopreserved. Ten of twelve cryopreserved oocytes survived after thawing and nine were fertilized and developed into good quality embryos which were transferred in three different cycles to a gestational carrier. A singleton pregnancy was achieved after the third transfer, resulting in the delivery of a healthy male. Surrogate motherhood is, however, not allowed in the majority of countries because of ethical concern. Porcu *et al.* (2008) reported the first delivery of healthy twins by a patient with bilateral ovariectomy for ovarian cancer who conceived using her own cryopreserved oocytes. Seven oocytes were retrieved before ovariectomy and were cryopreserved. After four years three oocytes were thawed. The survival rate of 100% as well as the fertilization and cleavage rate of 100% demonstrated that eggs may be safely stored for several years. The twin pregnancy went uneventfully to term. Thus, oocyte storage may be a concrete, pragmatic alternative also for oncological patients. The duration of oocyte storage does not seem to interfere with the oocytes' survival, as pregnancies occur even after several years of gamete cryopreservation in liquid nitrogen.

Despite the difficulties in evaluating the true efficiency of cryopreservation with slow freezing, taking together all the clinical data available so far, a rough estimate of five implantations per 100 thawed oocytes may be done. Table 2.1 summarizes the clinical results of slow freezing.

Table 2.1. Laboratory and clinical results of slow freezing cycles

	Protocol	Thawing cycles (n)	Thawed oocytes (n)	Survival (%)	Fertilization (%)	Pregnancy per transfer (%)	Implantation (%)	Thawed oocytes/pregnancy (mean)	Pregnancy/thawed oocytes (%)	Miscarriages (%)	Births/thawed oocytes (%)	Children (n)
Chen C., 1986	DMSO		40	80	83						1	2
Al-Hasani, 1987	DMSO – PROH + S 0.1 M	57	205	25	56							
van Uem, 1987	DMSO	2	28	25		50		28 (28/1)	3.6	0	1	1
Chen C., 1988	DMSO	7	50	76	71							
Diedrich 1988	DMSO	48	157	87	58	18		79 (157/2)	1.27	100	0	0
Tucker, 1996	PROH + S 0.1 M	8	81	24.7	65	60	23	27 (81/3)	3.7	100	0	0
Porcu, 1997	PROH + S 0.1 M	1	12	33	50	100	100	12 (12/1)	8.3	0	3	1
Antinori, 1998	PROH + S 0.1 M		335	56	33	100	100				0.3	
Nawroth, 1998	PROH + S 0.1 M	1	7	42.8		100	100	7 (7/1)	12.5	100		
Polak de Fried, 1998	PROH + S 0.1 M	1	10	30	66	100	50	10 (10/1)	10	0	10	1

Table 2.1. (cont.)

Protocol		Thawing cycles (n)	Thawed oocytes (n)	Survival (%)	Fertilization (%)	Pregnancy per transfer (%)	Implantation (%)	Thawed oocytes/pregnancy (mean)	Pregnancy/thawed oocytes (%)	Miscarriages (%)	Births/thawed oocytes (%)	Children (n)
Tucker, 1998a	PROH + S 0.1 M	19	311	24	51	33.3	21.4	62 (311/5)	1.6	0	0.3	2
Tucker, 1998b	PROH + S 0.2 M	1	29	10	66	100	50	29 (29/1)	3.4	0	3.4	1
Yang, 1998	PROH + S 0.2 M	1	6	33	100	100	100	6 (6/1)	17			
Young, 1998	PROH + S 0.1 M	1	8	100	100	100	60	8 (8/1)	12.5	50		2
Porcu, 1999a	PROH + S 0.2 M		10	70						0		2
Wurfel, 1999		1	4	75	75	100	66	4 (4/1)	25	0	25	2
Chia, 2000	PROH + S 0.2 M	1	12	83	70	100	33	12 (12/1)	8.3	100	0	0
Porcu, 2000a	PROH + S 0.1 M	112	1502	54	57.7	14.2	14	94 (1502/16)	1	44	0.7	11
Porcu, 2001	PROH + S 0.1 M	4		64	59							4
Winslow, 2001		45	324	68.5	80.8	26.2	13.5	29 (324/11)	3.4	17	4.9	16
Chen SU, 2002	PROH + S 0.3 M	1	8	100	57	100	50	8 (8/1)	12.5	0	12.5	2

Study	Condition											
Porcu, 2002	PROH + S 0.1 M	206	12	76	59	24.2	25	18 (109/6)	5.5	67		
Quintans, 2002	Na depleted	109		63		50					1.8	2
Yang, 2002	PROH + S 0.2 M	158	24	71	86.4	45.8	25.3	14 (158/11)	7			14
Boldt, 2003	0.2 M sucrose, Na depleted medium	90	16	74.4	59	36	20	22 (90/4)	4.4	0	5.5	5
Fosas, 2003	PROH + S 0.3 M	88	7	89.8	73.4	57.1	25	22 (88/4)	5.6	0	5.6	5
Huttelova, 2003	PROH + S 0.1 M	38	7	89.5	73.5	33		38 (38/1)	2.6	0	2.6	1
Notrica, 2003	PROH + S 0.1 M	14		57							1	
Allan, 2004	PROH + S 0.1 M	36		50				36 (36/1)	2.8	100	0	
Borini, 2004	PROH + S 0.2 M	737	68	37	45.4	25.4	16.4	49 (737/15)	2	20	1.5	13
Miller, 2004	PROH + S 0.1 M	12	1	100	75	100	50	12 (12/1)	8.3			
Azambuja, 2005	Na depleted	8	1	63	80	100	25	8 (8/1)	12.5	0	12.5	1
Chen SU, 2005	PROH + S 0.3 M	159	21	75	67	33	11	23 (159/7)	4.4	16.7	2.5	5

Table 2.1. (cont.)

	Protocol	Thawing cycles (n)	Thawed oocytes (n)	Survival (%)	Fertilization (%)	Pregnancy per transfer (%)	Implantation (%)	Thawed oocytes/ pregnancy (mean)	Pregnancy/ thawed oocytes (%)	Miscarriages (%)	Births/ thawed oocytes (%)	Children (n)
Li, 2005	PROH + S 0.3 M	12	81	90	83	47	10	20 (81/4)	5	25	7.4	3
Porcu, 2005			2750	69.6	73.9	17	10.1	32 (2750/85)	3	28	2.5	70
Tjer, 2005	PROH + S 0.3 M	1	14	71	80	100	50	14 (14/1)	7.1	0	7.1	1
Boldt, 2006	Na depleted	46	361	60.4	62	32.6	13.6	26 (361/14)	3.8			9
Borini, 2006a	PROH + S 0.1 M		918	43	51.5	19.2	12.3	66 (918/14)	1.5		0.6	12
Borini, 2006b	PROH + S 0.3 M	201	927	74	76	9.7	5.2	52 (927/18)	2	14.2	0.4	4
Chamayou, 2006	PROH + S 0.3 M		337	78			2				0.6	2
De Santis, 2006	PROH + S 0.3 M	68	396	71	80.4	9.5	5.7	66 (396/6)	1.5	33	0.25	2
De Santis, 2006	PROH + S 0.1 M	65	506	24	53.5	16.7	12.2	101 (506/5)	1	40	0.4	1
La Sala, 2006	PROH + S 0.3 M	518	1647	73	74.7	4.2	6.3	57 (1647/29)	1.76	47.4	0.42	7
Levi Setti, 2006	PROH + S 0.3 M	159	1087	69.9	67.5	12.4	5.7	60 (1087/18)	1.7	33.3	1.1	13
Montag, 2006	PROH + S 0.2 M	1	12	42	60	100	33	12 (12/1)	8.3	0	8.3	1

Study											
Noyes, 2006	9	137	93	89	44	27	35 (137/4)	2.9			
Baritt, 2007 PROH+S 0.3 M	4	79	86	89.7	75	26.1	26 (79/3)	3.80			
Bianchi, 2007 PROH+S 0.2 M	90	403	76	82.5	21.3	19	24 (403/17)	4.2	11.8	1	4
Borini, 2007a PROH+S 0.3 M	660	3238	68.1	76.1	14.9	15.5	9(3238/355)	11	21.9	1.7	60
Borini, 2007b									23		105
De Geyter, 2007 DMSO+PROH	15	73	60.8	72.7	33	12.5	24 (73/3)	4.1	66	1.4	1
Gook, 2007a PROH+S 0.2 M		6	67	25	100	100	6(6/1)	17	0	16	1
Konc, 2007 PROH+S 0.3 M	25	87	80	81	24	13.5	15 (87/6)	7	16	2.3	3
Yang, 2007 PROH+S 0.2 M	3	12	83.3	90	33	11.1	12 (12/1)	8.3	50	8.3	1
Ding, 2008									33		3
Konc, 2008a PROH+S 0.3 M	54	215	80	84	24	11	16 (215/13)	6	23	2.8	7
Konc, 2008b PROH+S 0.3 M	29	110	76	76	24	15.4	16 (110/7)	6.4	14	5.5	7
Parmegiani, 2008 PROH+S 0.3 M	93	437	75.1	86	19.3	9.6	27(437/16)	3.7	31.3	2.5	11

Table 2.1. (cont.)

Protocol		Thawing cycles (n)	Thawed oocytes (n)	Survival (%)	Fertilization (%)	Pregnancy per transfer (%)	Implantation (%)	Thawed oocytes/ pregnancy (mean)	Pregnancy/ thawed oocytes (%)	Miscarriages (%)	Births/ thawed oocytes (%)	Children (n)
Porcu, 2008												2
Borini, 2010	PROH + S 0.3 M	940	5076	55.5	72.5	17	10.1	39 (5076/ 129)	2.5	27.9	1.7	88
Smith, 2010	PROH + S 0.3 M	30	238	67	67	21	9.5	60 (238/4)	1.7	20	2.5	6
Azambuja, 2011	Na depleted	159		57.4	67.2	37.7	14.5			21		42
Virant-Klun, 2011	PROH + S 0.3 M	23	166	70.5	61.5	33.3		42 (166/4)	2.4	0	2.4	4
Bianchi, 2012	PROH + S 0.3 M	443	2458	71.8	77.9	22.8	13.5	27 (2458/90)	3.7	35.5	3.1	77

In the general awakening of interest about oocyte cryopreservation, the late 1990s also saw the resurgence of attention towards vitrification as an alternative technique for storing human eggs. Vitrification was originally proposed by Rall and Fahy (1985) in mouse embryos. Unlike slow freezing, the application of vitrification techniques to human oocytes occurred in the absence of basic biological studies addressing safety issues. Kuleshova et al. (1999) obtained the first birth, of a healthy girl, from vitrified human oocytes and reported an egg survival rate of 65%. This survival rate was not higher than that achieved in slow freezing. However, vitrification appeared attractive as potentially it would avoid the development of ice crystals and would be a simpler and cheaper technique. The most important variables that influence the results of vitrification are the choice of cryoprotectants, the exposure time, the prefreezing temperature and the devices for storing samples in liquid nitrogen. Several modifications have been introduced to improve the efficiency of the technique including increasing the cooling rates and the cryoprotectant concentration and reducing cryoprotectant toxicity. The cooling rate can be increased by reducing the volume of the cryoprotectant solution and directly exposing the biological sample to liquid nitrogen in either an open straw or an electron microscopy grid. A very high concentration of ethylene glycol (EG; 5.5 M) and sucrose (1.0 M) apparently displayed very low toxicity (Kuleshova et al., 1999). Using the same cryoprotectant solution in combination with grids achieved a pregnancy from immature human oocytes (Wu et al., 2001) and seven births from mature oocytes (Yoon et al., 2003) with an oocyte survival rate, respectively, of 59% and 69%. Kim et al. (2003, 2005) achieved, respectively, one pregnancy and four births by using Kuleshova's cryoprotectant solution. Ruvalcaba et al. (2005) obtained the birth of five children. Chian et al. (2005) used an especially designed device (Cryoleaf) and obtained a 93.9% survival rate, 74.6% fertilization rate and seven pregnancies. Another type of vitrification device is the Cryotop, which was designed by Kuwayama et al. (2005); with this device and a slightly lower concentration of EG (5.0 M) these authors obtained a 91% egg survival rate and 90% fertilization rate. Cobo et al. (2008c) published the birth of a healthy boy in a donation cycle. The births of an additional 28 children in 57 ovum donation cycles were also reported (Cobo et al., 2008b). In this study, oocyte survival rate was 96.1% and fertilization rate was 73.1%. In a further study (Cobo et al., 2008c), a comparison between fresh and vitrified oocytes was carried out in terms of survival, fertilization, cleavage, pregnancy and implantation rates. When evaluated simultaneously, the potential of vitrified oocytes to be fertilized and further develop was similar to that of fresh counterparts, with a survival rate of 96.9%, a fertilization rate around 76.3% and 11 ongoing pregnancies.

A different vitrification protocol with 2.7 M EG + 2.1 M DMSO + 0.5 M sucrose also resulted in pregnancies and births (Katayama et al., 2003; Kyono et al., 2005; Okimura et al., 2005; Lucena et al., 2006; Selman et al., 2006; Antinori et al., 2007). One more vitrification protocol, the super rapid cooling using slush nitrogen (SN2), was recently introduced. By applying negative pressure with a vacuum, liquid nitrogen will freeze and will be transformed into a slush state (SN2), which avoids the development of gas bubbles when plunging a biological sample. With this vitrification strategy, Yoon et al. (2007) achieved an 85.1% survival rate (302 out of 364 frozen eggs), 77.4% fertilization rate, 94.3% cleavage rate and 13 pregnancies (43.3%) from 30 uterine transfers of 120 embryos.

Studies on oocyte vitrification after in vitro maturation of immature oocytes have also been carried out. Huang et al. (2007b) reported the successful vitrification of three in vitro matured oocytes as a strategy of fertility preservation in women with borderline ovarian malignancy. The same author (Huang et al., 2008b) published the results of four cryopreservation cycles after in vitro maturation. After achieving a mean maturation rate of 79%, a total of eight oocytes were vitrified. In the authors' opinion, this technique seems to be associated with satisfying fertilization rates (Huang *et al.*, 2008b).

The first live birth of a healthy baby after vitrification of in vitro matured oocytes was recently reported (Chian *et al.*, 2008).

Until recently, just over 60 births from oocyte vitrification had been published. Then, suddenly, the births of another 200 children were reported (Chian *et al.*, 2008). Rather unusually, the paper did not report details on the number of warming cycles; the number of vitrified-warmed oocytes; the egg survival, fertilization and cleavage rates and the pregnancy rate. Vitrification medium composed of 15% EG and PROH or 15% EG and DMSO, plus 0.5 M sucrose were used. The oocytes were then loaded onto the McGill Cryoleaf or Cryotop and directly immersed into liquid nitrogen. Obstetric and perinatal outcomes of 165 pregnancies and 200 infants conceived with vitrified oocytes were evaluated. The multiple pregnancy rate was 17%. The mean gestational age was 37 weeks + 1 day, the preterm deliveries (34–37 weeks) were 30% and the early preterm delivery (<34 weeks) rates were 6%. The mean birth weight was 2920 ± 37 g for singletons and 2231 ± 55 g for multiples. The incidence of congenital anomalies was 2.5%. These results indicate that the mean birth weight and the incidence of congenital anomalies are comparable to those of spontaneous conceptions.

A few studies have addressed the issue of meiotic spindle integrity in human oocytes after vitrification. Noyes *et al.* (2006) established an association between the presence of the meiotic spindle after thawing and warming and the subsequent development of competent embryos. Larman *et al.* (2007b) documented the maintenance of the meiotic spindle during vitrification in human and mouse oocytes. Ciotti *et al.* (2009) investigated the behavior of the meiotic spindle during vitrification and demonstrated that meiotic spindle recovery is faster in vitrification of human oocytes than with slow freezing. These data support a possible protective effect of vitrification on the meiotic spindle structure and, therefore, on the subsequent clinical outcome of the procedure, although additional basic biological studies as well as comparative clinical studies are needed.

To date, it is still difficult to assess the true efficacy of egg storage in ART as sufficient consistency and reproducibility of results are still to be achieved. The considerable variability in implantation rates per thawed or warmed oocyte is due more to the patient population, clinical conditions, oocyte quality and number of embryos transferred than to the cryopreservation technique itself. Slow freezing seems to produce results apparently less favorable than those obtained with vitrification. Nevertheless, it must be taken into consideration that the largest series of egg slow freezing have been performed in Italy where the insemination of no more than three eggs is allowed. In these studies, oocyte freezing is used in the general ART population and therefore also in cases with less favorable prognosis. On the other hand, most papers on vitrification included selected populations, frequently with donor programs, very young patients and a very large number of embryos transferred. Table 2.2 summarizes the clinical results of oocyte vitrification.

Safety of oocyte cryopreservation

As regards safety, the first report that evaluated this aspect of oocyte cryopreservation was published by Porcu *et al.* (2000a). Results regarding 17 pregnancies obtained from oocytes that had been cryopreserved were reported in terms of obstetric complications, perinatal

Table 2.2. Laboratory and clinical results of human oocyte vitrification

	Protocol (device)	Thawing cycles (n)	Thawed oocytes (n)	Survival (%)	Fertilization (%)	Pregnancy (%)	Implantation (%)	Thawed oocytes/ pregnancy (mean)	Pregnancy/ thawed oocytes (%)	Miscarriages (%)	Births/ thawed oocytes (%)	Children (n)
Kuleshova, 1999	EG 5.5 M + S 1.0 M (OPS)	4	17	65	45	33	33	17 (17/1)	5.8	0	5.8	1
Wu, 2001	EG 5.5 M + S 1.0 M (Grids)	36	79	59	70	33	50	79 (79/1)	1.3			
Katayama, 2003	EG 2.7 M + S 0.5 M + DMSO 2.1 M (Cryotop)	6	46	94	91	33	20	23 (46/2)	4.3	50	2.1	1
Kim, 2003	EG 5.5 M + S 1.0 M (Grids)	3	51	80	54	33						
Yoon, 2003	EG 5.5 M + S 1.0 M (Grids)	34	474	68.6	71.7	21.4	6.4	79 (474/6)	1.3	0	1.5	7
Chian, 2005	EG + PROH + S 0.5 M (Cryoleaf)	15	180	94	74.6	46.7	20.4	26 (180/7)	4			
Kim, 2005	EG 5.5 M + S 1.0 M (Grids)	10	186	74.7	55.2	40	15.3	46.5 (186/4)	2	50	4.3	4
Kuwayama, 2005	EG 5.0 M + S 1.0 M (Cryotop)		64	91	90			5.3 (64/12)	18.8			7

Table 2.2. (cont.)

Protocol (device)	Thawing cycles (n)	Thawed oocytes (n)	Survival (%)	Fertilization (%)	Pregnancy (%)	Implantation (%)	Thawed oocytes/pregnancy (mean)	Pregnancy/thawed oocytes (%)	Miscarriages (%)	Births/thawed oocytes (%)	Children (n)
Kyono, 2005	EG 2.7 M + S 0.5 M + DMSO 2.1 M (Cryotop)	1	5	100	66	100	100	5 (5/1)	20	0	20	1
Okimura, 2005	EG 2.7 M + S 0.5 M + DMSO 2.1 M (Cryotop)		64	91	89.6	41.4	20	5.3 (64/12)	18.8	17	11	7
Ruvalcaba, 2005		10	60	76.6	82.6	80	32.3	7.5 (60/8)	13.3	50	7	5
Lucena, 2006	EG 2.7 M + S 0.5 M + DMSO 2.1 M (Cryotop)	23	159	75	87.2	56.5	20	12 (159/13)	8.2			
Selman, 2006	EG 2.7 M + S 0.5 M + DMSO 2.1 M (OPS)	6	24	75	77.7	33.3	21.4	12 (24/2)	8.3			
Smith, 2006	EG 5.0 M + S 1.0 M (Cryotop)	10		80	83	55						
Antinori, 2007	EG 2.7 M + S 0.5 M + DMSO 2.1 M (Cryotop)	120	330	99	93	32.5	13	8.4 (330/39)	11.8	20.5	1	3

Yoon, 2007	SN 2 (Gold grids)	30	364	85.1	77.4	43.3	14.2	28 (364/13)	3.6	15.4	1	5
Chang, 2008	EG 15%+DMSO 15%+S 0.5 M (Cryotop)	2	18	100	89	50	33	9 (18/2)	11	0		
Chang, 2008a	EG 15%+DMSO 15%+S 0.5 M (Cryotop)	18	137	85	86	83.3	61.9	9.1 (137/15)	10.9	0	7.3	19
Chian, 2008												
Cobo, 2008a	EG 5.0 M+S 1.0 M (Cryotop)	1	5	80	50	100	50	5 (5/1)	20	50		200
Cobo, 2008b	EG 5.0 M+S 1.0 M (Cryotop)	57	693	96.1	73.1	63.2		19 (693/36)	5			28
Cobo, 2008c	EG+DMSO (Cryotop)	30	250	96.9	76.3	47.8	40.8	16.7 (250/15)	6	20	4.4	

OPS = open pulled straw.

outcomes and follow-up of children. These preliminary observations gave a first reassurance about the health of babies born. Eleven pregnancies out of seventeen ended with the delivery of 13 healthy children (9 females and 4 males). The amniocentesis performed in all but one pregnancy showed a normal karyotype. Obstetric complications registered were: two preterm deliveries, one placenta previa, and one instance of gestational hypertension. Mean gestational age at birth was 260 ± 17 days and mean birth weight was 2730 ± 537 g. The mean Apgar score at 5 minutes was 7.9 ± 0.9. No malformations were detected in the newborns. Cesarean section was performed in nine cases. Follow-up of the children showed a normal physical and cognitive development in all of them. These positive observations were confirmed in subsequent studies conducted on 70 children (Porcu, 2005) and 105 babies (Borini *et al.*, 2007a). In the latter, 149 pregnancies had brought to birth 105 babies, 73 in single pregnancies and 32 in twin pregnancies, with a 23% miscarriage rate. The mean gestational age at birth was 38.9 weeks and the mean birth weight was 3.353 g in singletons and 2.599 g in twins.

Recently, data regarding a very large population of 936 babies born after oocyte cryopreservation have been published (Noyes *et al.*, 2009). The authors built a database including all verified live-born infants between 1986 and 2008. Fifty-eight reports, which included 609 live-born babies (308 from slow freezing, 289 from vitrification and 12 from both methods), were reviewed. An additional 327 live births were documented (Table 2.3).

The rate of birth anomalies was found to be 1.3% (12), which is comparable with that in spontaneous pregnancies. The anomalies observed were: three ventricular septal defects,

Table 2.3. Data from oocyte cryopreservation births "series reports." (n = 35 reports: 23 slow freezing, 9 vitrification, 3 both cryopreservation methods)

Parameter	Cryopreservation method		
	Slow freeze	**Vitrification**	**Both**
No. of embryo transfers	*1974*	*834*	*19*
No. of oocytes thawed/ warmed	11 890	5435	271
No. of oocytes survived	*8056*	*4392*	*244*
% oocyte survival	68 (range: 22–90)	81 (range: 69–99)	90
% 2-pronucleate fertilization	*73 (range: 50–86)*	*79 (range: 59–93)*	*81*
No. of live born babies	282	285	12
Baby gender (information available for 168 slow freeze, 189 vitrification and 12 both methods)	*99 female, 69 male*	*86 female, 103 male*	*8 female, 4 male*
Birth defects	1 ventricular septal defect, 1 choanal atresia, 1 Rubinstein–Taybi syndrome	2 ventricular septal defects, 1 biliary atresia, 1 clubfoot, 1 skin hemangioma	None

Produced, with permission, from Noyes *et al.*, 2009.

Table 2.4. Birth anomalies in natural conception versus ooyte cryopreservation, listed most common to most rare

Birth anomaly	Approximate incidence in natural conception births	Incidence in total of 936 oocyte cryopreservation births (n)
All	One in 33	12 (one in 78)
Skin hemangioma	One in 50–225	1
Cardiac defects	One in 125	3
Neural tube defects	One in 385	0
Cleft lip and palate	One in 710	1
Clubfoot	One in 735	3
Arnold–Chiari syndrome	One in 1200	1
Choanal atresia	One in 7000	1
Biliary atresia	One in 10 000–15 000	1
Rubinsten–Taybi syndrome	One in 100 000–125 000	1

Produced, with permission, from Noyes et al., 2009.

one choanal and one biliary atresia, one Rubinstein–Taybi syndrome, one Arnold–Chiari syndrome, one cleft palate, three clubfoot and one skin haemangioma (Table 2.4).

Birth weight, gestational age and prematurity cannot be correctly evaluated in this study, because the parameters are not expressed separately for single and multiple births, as the authors underline. However, the rate of multiple gestations was 19%. The mean gestational age and weight at birth of the 30 babies reported in case reports were, respectively, 36.9 ± 0.6 weeks and 2720 ± 116 g in the slow freezing group and 39 ± 1 week and 3318 ± 201 g in the vitrification group.

These results are comparable with those achieved by Chian et al. (2008) who reported the obstetric and perinatal outcomes of 200 infants born in 165 pregnancies from oocyte vitrification. The multiple birth rate was 17% (26 twins and 2 triplets). The Cesarean section rate was 37% in singleton pregnancies and 96% in multiple pregnancies, whilst the mean birth weight was 2920 ± 37 g for singletons and 2231 ± 55 g for multiples. The incidence of congenital malformations was 2.5% (two ventricular septal defects, one biliary atresia, one club foot and one skin haemangioma) (Chian et al., 2008) (Table 2.5).

Another review of published data concerning live births after oocyte cryopreservation has been published by Wennerholm et al. (2009) who collected neonatal information about 148 children born from oocyte slow freezing and 221 children born after vitrification of oocyte. Although data were very limited, the birth weight of children conceived through oocyte cryopreservation were within the normal range.

On the whole, very limited data have been reported on pregnancy outcomes after oocyte cryopreservation, so further studies are necessary to evaluate the characteristics of

Table 2.5. Obstetric and perinatal outcomes and incidence of congenital malformations in children conceived after oocyte vitrification

Characteristics	All pregnancies (n = 165)	Singleton pregnancies (n = 137)	Multiple gestation pregnancies (n = 28)
Mean gestational age (weeks + days)	37 + 1	37 + 3	35 + 5
No of deliveries at 34–37 weeks (%)	46 (30)	30 (22)	16 (57)
No of deliveries at <34 weeks (%)	10 (6)	6 (4)	4 (14)
	All newborns (n = 200)	**Singleton newborns (n = 141)**	**Multiple gestation newborns (n = 59)**
Birth weight (mean +/− SEM) (g)	2784 +/− 37	2920 +/− 37	2231 +/− 55
No of LBW (%)	68 (34)	24 (17)	44 (74)
No of VLBW (%)	4 (2)	1 (0.7)	3 (5)
Median Apgar score at 1 min	8	9	8
Median Apgar score at 5 min	10	10	10
Incidence of congenital anomalies			
Biliary atresia	1	0	1
Clubfoot	1	1	0
Skin hemangioma	1	1	0
Ventricular septal defect	2	0	2
Total (%)	5 (2.5%)	2 (1.4)	3 (5.1)

LBW = low birth weight, 1500–2500 g; VLBW = very low birth weight, < 1500 g.
SEM = standard error of mean.
Produced, with permission, from Chian *et al.*, 2008.

pregnancies and the long-term follow-up of the children. The need is particularly urgent because of the experimental connotations of this technique. In order to follow up the outcomes and evaluate the efficacy and safety of oocyte cryopreservation techniques, a registry was recently adopted in the United States as a national five-year prospective, multicenter, observational study (HOPE: "The Human Oocyte Preservation Experience") (Ezcurra *et al.*, 2009).

Chapter 3

Clinical management
of oocyte cryopreservation

Ovarian stimulation and oocyte storage

Multiple ovulation induction is a clinical practice dating back to the first years of assisted reproduction, when we believed that many oocytes were needed to increase the chance of pregnancy. Several oocytes were used to obtain embryos for immediate transfer or to be frozen, an option that has ethical issues associated with it. As an alternative, oocytes may be harvested and stored in liquid nitrogen for future use, an option which does not raise ethical problems.

However, as the human species is essentially mono-ovulatory, multiple ovulation is not easy to achieve. Multiple ovulation induction methods are based on the use of high quantities of gonadotropins, which increase the number of follicles recruited and stimulate their maturation. The aim is to obtain as many synchronously mature follicles as possible, prevent their dehiscence and harvest oocytes surgically. Obtaining good quality oocytes is essential since they are the basis for the success of immediate embryo insemination or oocyte cryopreservation.

Obtaining good quality mature oocytes depends first on patient characteristics and, second, on the stimulation protocol. Whatever the stimulation protocol used, there is much less likelihood of obtaining numerous good quality oocytes suitable for cryopreservation from women over 40, with ovarian adenomyosis, or with initial precocious ovarian failure.

Storage of surplus eggs in a standard cycle

Cryopreservation is particularly suitable for oocytes from women under 38 years old with normal ovarian function. In this case, a stimulation protocol must foresee the initial administration of 225 IU recombinant gonadotropins for six days, in a cycle of hypophyseal desensitization obtained with a daily or depot gonadotropin-releasing hormone (GnRH) agonist. Subsequently, gonadotropin therapy must be modulated on the basis of the estrogenic and follicle response. Generally, dosages are not increased and are rarely reduced.

On average, stimulation time is 12 days and the number of mature follicles is 10. Final maturity induction and follicular breakage are obtained with 10 000 IU of human chorionic gonadotropin (HCG). Transvaginal ultrasound-guided follicle aspiration is carried out after 36 hours. Each follicle undergoes careful curettage to obtain as many oocytes as possible. Follicle flushing is not required. Subsequently, the oocytes must be kept at 37 °C and examined rapidly in order to evaluate their quality and maturity after denudation and PolsCope observation. The average number of cryopreservable excess oocytes among these patients is five. Oocytes must be cryopreserved within four hours from recovery.

Egg storage to avoid ovarian hyperstimulation syndrome

The risk of developing ovarian hyperstimulation syndrome (OHSS) during superovulation cycles is 1–2%. Ovarian hyperstimulation syndrome represents a potentially lethal iatrogenic complication in PMA techniques. The literature shows an incidence of 1–10% in PMA cycles; the most serious forms appear in 0.5–2%. The triggering event is the outflow of vasoactive substances generated as a consequence of HCG administration. This provokes excessive transfer of liquid from the intravascular compartment to the interstitial space.

The symptomatology regresses in the absence of pregnancy. On the contrary, in the case of pregnancy, the case history could seriously get worse, even leading to death, and, in any case, requiring hospitalization, with a notable impact on public health expenses. In recent years, several techniques for minimizing these complications among patients at risk have been suggested, such as suspension of the stimulation cycle or the use of a GnRH antagonist or eliminating HCG administration. Currently, one of the most common procedures used in PMA centers is embryo transfer only after remission of the clinical symptomatology. This requires embryo freezing until transfer is possible.

Studies have shown the effectiveness of these procedures in reducing the risk of developing OHSS with brilliant results in terms of pregnancy on postponed transfer cycles of frozen embryos. The disadvantage is that a large number of cryopreserved embryos have to be discarded. Oocyte cryopreservation is an alternative option to embryo preservation, leading to postponement of fertilization and embryo transfer until the next cycle. This procedure prevents any potential lethal clinical conditions and permits the conservation of biological material without any ethical and legal problems, unlike embryo freezing.

Stimulation cycles considered at risk for OHSS present with more than 10 small follicles (diameter less than 12 mm) and estradiol levels up to 3000 pg/ml. OHSS usually occurs in young women with polycystic ovaries, patients with past OHSS or sometimes in women without any particular predisposition in their medical history or hormone profile. For the cases at risk, stimulation is modulated through the reduction of gonadotropin dosage, continuing administration in order to obtain some mature follicles. The dosage of HCG (5000 IU) is reduced. In that way, the risk of severe OHSS is limited. The subsequent follicle aspiration leads to the recovery of an average of 15 oocytes that can be cryopreserved.

In such patients, the post-pickup course is usually favorable. The need for hospital care is reduced to 2 ± 2 days and there is a low incidence of ascites, and hemoconcentration and hemocoagulative alterations.

Hematological and echographic parameters should be examined after one week, with the pharmacological preparation of the endometrium scheduled for the following month. The effects of oocyte thawing, insemination and developed embryo implantation are particularly favorable. This technique does not reduce fertilization capability and it prevents severe OHSS complications. The results are comparable to those obtained with elective cryopreservation of all the embryos in the same clinical conditions.

Egg storage in polycystic ovary syndrome

Polycystic ovary syndrome (PCOS) is a well-known dysfunctional clinical condition which can sometimes impair fertility. Superovulation management can be rather difficult even if PCOS is not the cause of infertility but there are male problems or tubal and idiopathic complications. A polycystic ovary is particularly sensitive to gonadotropin stimulation.

While at the beginning, it may give feedback which is too slow and unsuitable; later, it could cause a surplus of follicles at different stages of maturity with a preponderance of small follicles. These are the presuppositions for the risk of multiple pregnancies in case of intrauterine insemination (IUI) and the risk of developing OHSS.

In PCOS patients oocyte cryopreservation offers a solution for salvaging the treatment cycle without any suspension. Ovarian stimulation must be carried out very carefully in order to reduce the risk of OHSS and produce good quality oocytes for future cryopreservation. Our protocol of ovulation induction uses initial dosages of recombinant follicle-stimulating hormone (FSH) of no more than 150 IU/day. To control the early luteinizing hormone (LH) surge, we administer a GnRH antagonist (cetrorelix or ganirelix) as soon as the follicle reaches 14 mm. When the follicular development is completed, we administrate a reduced dosage of HCG (5000 IU) in order to limit the risk of OHSS development. The withdrawal of the oocytes is carried out after 36 hours, as usual.

If OHSS risk is moderate, it is possible to continue with the elective insemination of only two oocytes and the cryopreservation of the surplus oocytes. On the contrary, if the risk of OHSS is severe, the only thing to do is to cryopreserve all the oocytes collected. In the case of IUI with excessive follicular development, it is possible to retrieve the oocytes and freeze them until ovary normalization. In patients with a polycystic ovary, even when there is not a severe risk of OHSS, we usually recruit a large number of oocytes to be cryopreserved in some measure. Asynchrony of oocyte development is frequently responsible for immature oocyte recovery. Currently, the cryopreservation of immature oocytes does not seem to be useful in clinical terms.

Generally, 70% of the oocytes collected from a polycystic ovary can be cryopreserved. The ovarian quality is good and freezing survival of the oocytes is approximately 80%. Fertilization and cleavage are satisfactory as are the results in terms of pregnancy. It is interesting to point out the high pregnancy rate per patient, which is related to the possibility of doing subsequent embryo transfers obtained from a large number of frozen oocytes after a unique follicle aspiration.

Egg storage in cancer patients

Development of antineoplastic therapies has led to a gradual increase in the survival rate in cancer patients and particular attention has been paid to the potential fertility damage caused by antiblastic or surgical therapies in these patients. It is extremely important to work out solutions capable of protecting fertilization in these patients. Cryopreservation of ovarian tissue is one option; however, this presents the risk of reintroducing neoplastic cells with the reimplantation procedure. Embryo cryopreservation is another option for obviating impaired fertility as is oocyte cryopreservation (which is one of the most recent procedures and has less ethical and legal problems).

Ovulation induction must be carried out in oocyte or embryo cryopreservation; in this case, it is essential to avoid damage endangering the patient by stimulating neoplastic growth or recurrence.

Therapeutic protocols must be planned, taking into consideration the urgency of antiblastic therapy and the cycle stage before starting. The choice is between a flare-up protocol with a combination of a GnRH agonist and gonadotropins beginning on the first day of the month or a long protocol with desensitization by a GnRH agonist followed by stimulation with gonadotropin. For hypophysial desensitization, some protocols include the use of a GnRH agonist while others use GnRH antagonists. Protocols usually foresee the use of recombinant FSH and seldom use urinary FSH.

Porcu *et al.* (2004) reported the results of treating 18 patients affected by extragynecological neoplasms (lymphoma and leukemia, predominantly). Ovarian stimulation allowed the recovery and cryopreservation of an average of 15 oocytes without any secondary consequences or complications, such as OHSS. The choice of therapy depends on potential neoplasm hormone-sensitivity.

During ovarian induction, high levels of circulating estrogen can be achieved. In the case of an estrogen-sensitive cancer, these could enhance the neoplasm or induce a potential recurrence. In these cases, the combination of gonadotropins with aromatase inhibitors, such as letrozole, or with tamoxifen, paying particular attention to the serumal estradiol rate, has attained great results regarding the number of oocytes recovered, fertilization rate and the number of embryos developed. Cases of recurrence among oncology patients are not significant. However, it is essential to carry out additional research, to increase the number of patients and to lengthen the follow-up period.

Many authors have evaluated the effects of assisted reproduction in patients affected by endometrial cancer, who were treated with early progestinic therapy. Before starting progestinic therapy, all patients undergo histological diagnosis through curettage and cancer staging using magnetic resonance and levels of serum CA-125 in order to preclude invasion of the myometrium or metastasis at a distance. Although there are no standard therapeutic regimes, progestinic therapy foresees the use of high dosages of megestrole acetate (at least 160 mg/day for 6 months or 400 mg/day for 3 months). As soon as at least two bioptic endometrial samples are negative, patients start to receive assisted fertilization treatment.

Elizur *et al.* (2007) investigated the effects of medically assisted fertilization cycles carried out on eight patients who had previously been treated with progestinic therapy for endometrial cancer. For some of them, a flare-up protocol was used; for the others, a long protocol with a GnRH agonist was used. A GnRH antagonist was used in only one cycle. For ovarian stimulation, 225 IU/die of human menopausal gonadotropins (HMG) or recombinant FSH were used. Stimulation took 10 days, on average. Endometrial thickness never exceeded 10 mm in any patient. With regard to neoplasm recurrence rate, some studies have not shown any recurrence 2–4 months after the birth. On the contrary, in Elizur's study, three of the eight patients, under medical treatment, had a recurrence.

Ovarian induction of ovulation is generally associated with good results (Table 3.1) in women affected by borderline ovarian cancer who undergo conservative surgery. Among studies on cool embryo transfer in patients with borderline ovarian cancer, Fasouliotis *et al.*'s (2004) study reported an average of eight oocytes recovered; six of the eight were mature with a fertilization rate of 57%. The average number of embryos transferred was three, the pregnancy rate per oocyte retrieval was 37%, while the pregnancy rate per transfer was 43%. All children were in good health. Park *et al.*'s (2007) study showed an average of six oocytes recovered, with a fertilization rate of 74%, a clinical pregnancy rate of 50%, an implantion rate of 32% and a live birth rate of 50%. Elizur's results showed an average of nine oocytes recovered, a fertility rate of 59%, a pregnancy rate per cycle of 28% and pregnancy rate per transfer of 29%. Four of the eight patients (50%) gave birth to six newborns in good health (one of the patients had a trigeminal pregnancy).

Table 3.1. Results of ovulation induction in cancer patients

Study	Type of cancer	Type of protocol	No. patients	Average age (years)	Stimulation (days)	Estradiol (pg/ml)	Oocytes collected	Embryos/cycle	No. cycles IVF	Clinical pregnancy/cycle	Follow-up (months)	Recurrence (%)
Porcu, 2004	Leukemia, lymphoma, sarcoma, Wilms' disease, craniopharyngioma	GnRH agonists + rFSH	18	19	11	978 ± 558	15 ± 6	0	18	–	–	–
Hoffman, 1999	Ovary (borderline)	GnRH agonists uFSH + rFSH	1	28	–	–	8 / 10	4 / 10	1 / 1	0 / 1/1	–	0
Attar, 2004	Ovary (borderline)	GnRH agonists + rFSH	1	29	–	675	3	2	1	1/1	9	0
Fasouliotis, 2004	Ovary (borderline)	GnRH agonists + rFSH	5	32	–	1493 ± 558	8	3	17	6/17	39	20
Park, 2007	Ovary (borderline)	GnRH agonists + rFSH	5	30	–	1033	6	–	13	6/13	30	0
Fortin, 2007	Ovary (borderline)	Clomiphene/rFSH	30	28	–	–	–	–	75	13/75	93	16
Porcu, 2008	Ovary (borderline)	GnRH agonists + rFSH	1	26	10	1750	7	3	1	1/1	39	0
Oktay, 2005	Breast	Tamoxifen / Tamoxifen + rFSH / Letrozole + rFSH	29	37 / 38 / 39	8 / 9 / 9	419 ± 39 / 1182 ± 271 / 380 ± 57	2 / 7 / 12	1 / 4 / 5	13 / 9 / 11	0	20 / 14 / 9	7 / 3 / 0
Oktay, 2006	Breast	Letrozole + GnRH agonists + rFSH	47	36	12	483 ± 278	12	7	47	1/3	–	–

Azim, 2007	Breast	Anastrozole + GnRH antag + rFSH	7	36	11	2515 ± 1368	10	6	–	9/16	–	–
		Letrozole + GnRH antag + rFSH	47	36	10	714 ± 441	12	6				
Azim, 2008	Breast	Letrozole + GnRH antag + rFSH	79	36	9.87	406 ± 257	10	6	–	4/5	23	4
Pinto, 2001	Endometrium	GnRH agonists + rFSH	1	29	–	–	11	7	1	0	4	0
						–	16	10	1	0		
						2621	36	29	1	1/1		
Yarali, 2004	Endometrium	GnRH agonists + rFSH	1	32	–	–	9	6	1	1/1	2	0
Azim, 2007	Endometrium	Letrozole + GnRH antag + rFSH	4	33	–	387 ± 103	7	5	5	1/5	30	0
Elizur 2007	Endometrium	GnRH agonists/ antag + hMG/rFSH	8	29	10	1203 ± 847	9	2	31	9/31	31	37

In a recent study, Porcu *et al.* (2008) reported the first birth after a medically assisted procreation cycle in a patient (affected by borderline ovarian cancer) who underwent bilateral ovariectomy and whose oocytes had been frozen for four years. Through ovarian stimulation, carried out before the ovariectomy, 15 oocytes were recovered and frozen without any complications. Three embryo transfers led to a bigeminal pregnancy. The newborns were healthy.

Among studies on frozen embryo cycles, carried out on breast cancer patients not undergoing any antiblastic treatment cycle, Oktay et al. (2006) reported an average of 12 oocytes recovered and an average of 7 embryos per cycle. Up to the publication date, only three patients had returned for embryo transfer. Only one of the three was pregnant and gave birth at 36 weeks' gestation. Azim *et al.*'s (2007a) study reported an average of 11 oocytes recovered. All embryos were frozen; the clinical pregnancy rate was 56% and the childbirth rate was 37%, with the result of six newborns who did not show any deformities. Azim's (2008) study reported an average of 10 oocytes recovered, with 6 embryo formations per cycle. All embryos generated (or oocytes in the absence of a partner) were cryopreserved. Ten patients returned to undergo embryo transfer. The result was eight pregnancies and five births (all the newborns were healthy). Azim and Oktay's (2007) study on four endometrial cancer patients, reported an average of seven oocytes, the generation of five embryos per cycle and a clinical pregnancy rate of 25% (trigeminal childbirth in the 31st week of gestation in a surrogate; the other three patients requested that their embryos be frozen).

It is extremely important to personalize a therapy on the basis of patient age, monitoring the reactions during treatment for ovarian cancer. This could avoid the risk of OHSS. In Elizur *et al.*'s (2007) study, ovulation induction treatment was interrupted in a patient at risk of developing OHSS. In conclusion, before we can undertake an ovulation induction therapy in cancer patients, it is essential to consider some variables: (1) patient age, (2) type of neoplasm and (3) timing for ovulation induction before antiblastic treatment.

Laboratory management of oocyte cryopreservation

The egg freezing laboratory: location, equipment, instruments, materials

The laboratory must be of dimensions adequate for the amount of work carried out by the center, located near the embryology laboratory, and furnished with the equipment and specific materials for cryopreservation.

The necessary equipment for a cryobiological laboratory includes:

- Laminar flow hood with stereomicroscope and hotplate (Figure 4.1)
- Thermostat
- CO_2 incubator
- Programmable freezer + pressure pump (Figures 4.2 and 4.3)
- Dewars room with dewars containing biological samples (Figure 4.4)
- Refrigerator at 4 °C (for freezing and thawing solutions).

Selecting freezable eggs: the freezable egg score

Selecting a freezable egg involves the following steps:

1. Evaluation of oocyte maturity and quality.
2. Grading of the oocyte.

Evaluation of oocyte maturity and quality

The oocyte is the female germinal cell. The characteristic of these cell lines is that of developing by means of a particular cell division mechanism called meiosis. This consists of two successive cell divisions which give origin to a cell with a genetic haploid patrimony, the female gamete.

During antral growth, after ovulation, the oocyte is surrounded by two types of granulosa cells: cells of the cumulus oophorus and those of the corona radiata. The former are more dispersed while the latter are in direct contact with the zona pellucida (ZP) and are anchored to it by extensions. Some of the latter push until they contact the plasmatic membrane of the oocyte, with which they establish "gap" junctions which permit metabolic cooperation between the various cells. Through these connections, the follicular cells can provide metabolic or regulating substances to the oocyte.

The cumulus oophorus, together with the egg cell, constitutes the cumulus-corona-oocyte complex (CCOC). Under the optic microscope, this structure assumes different morphological

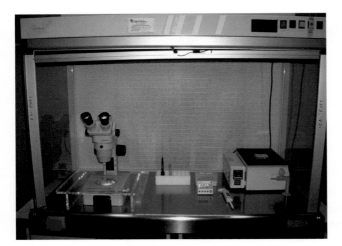

Figure 4.1 Laminar flow hood with stereomicroscope and hotplate.

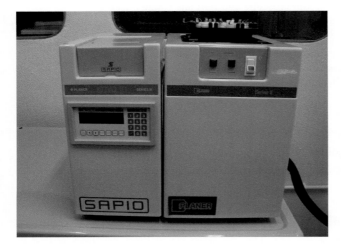

Figure 4.2 Programmable freezer.

characteristics according to the stage of maturation. For example, the preovulatory peak of gonadotropin also stimulates the cells of the cumulus, which, in response, produce a notable quantity of extracellular matrix predominantly made up of hyaluronic acid. This accumulates as a mucilaginous substance among the cells and causes their dissociation. Consequently, the morphology is modified because the cumulus increases its dimensions. This phenomenon is known as expansion or mucification of the cumulus.

During the collection of the oocytes of a stimulated cycle using a stereomicroscope, we can therefore observe different morphological pictures whose definition is obviously influenced by subjective variations:

Cumulus-enclosed oocyte (CEO): the oocyte is completely enclosed by cells of the cumulus. It is very small and difficult to identify except at the highest magnification of the stereomicroscope.

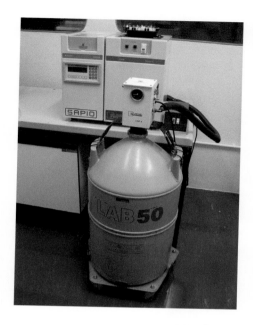

Figure 4.3 Programmable freezer connected to the pressure pump.

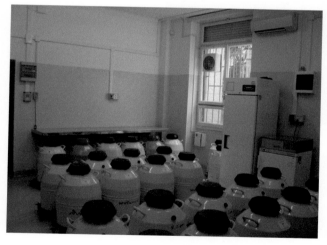

Figure 4.4 Room dedicated to dewars containing biological samples.

Very immature oocyte or germinal vesicle (prophase I): the cells of the cumulus and the corona are very compact and adhere tightly to the oocyte; the ooplasm is not often visible (Figure 4.5).

Immature oocyte (metaphase I): the cumulus oophorus is rather expanded, the cells of the corona are not completely expanded, and the ooplasm is visible, even if it is still slightly covered at the edges (Figure 4.6).

Mature oocyte (metaphase II): cumulus oophorus and corona radiata with expanded cells to form a characteristic radiating structure; the ooplasm, and sometimes also the first polar body (PB), are visible (Figure 4.7).

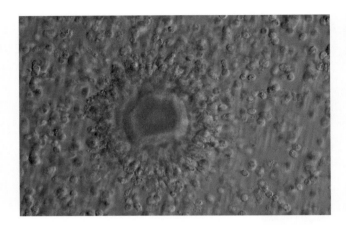

Figure 4.5 Very immature oocyte (prophase I): note the dark cumulus/corona cells near the oocyte and the dark ooplasm.

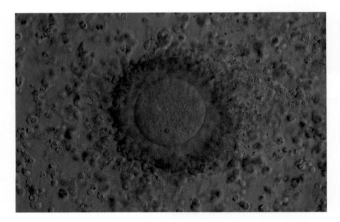

Figure 4.6 Immature oocyte (metaphase I). Compared to Figure 4.5, the cumulus cells are more expanded, the corona cells are dark and near the oocyte, the ooplasm is slightly dark.

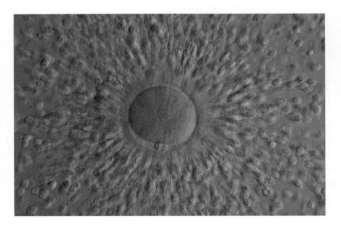

Figure 4.7 Mature oocyte (metaphase II). The cumulus/corona cells are clear and expanded to form the characteristic radial structure; the ooplasm has a clear color.

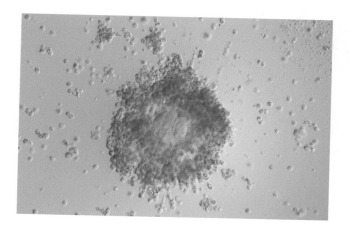

Figure 4.8 Post-mature oocyte. The cumulus/corona cells are dark and scattered and the ooplasm is dark.

Post-mature oocyte: the cells of the cumulus oophorus and the corona are unhomogeneously distributed, forming dark clusters which progressively detach from the oocyte (Figure 4.8).

Evaluation of cumulus-corona-oocyte complex maturity

Methodology

The contents of each sample of follicular liquid are poured into a Petri dish. The **CCOC** is identified by analyzing the follicular liquid at 6X magnification. By simply inclining the dish, a reduction in the thickness of the liquid in which it is found is obtained. In this way, the **CCOC** is outstretched on the bottom of the dish facilitating observation and evaluation of the maturity of the **CCOC**, which is carried out using maximum magnification (40X).

Evaluation of the nucleus

Evaluation of the nucleus can be done after oocyte denudation. The modality of enzymatic and mechanical removal of the cells of the cumulus and the corona is as follows: a 4 wells Nunclon (Nunclon, Nunk, Roskilde, Denmark) is prepared by filling one well with 0.5 ml of hyaluronidase (Cook IVF, Brisbane, Australia) diluted to a final concentration of 40 IU/ml and the other three wells with 0.5 ml Fertilization Medium (Cook IVF, Brisbane, Australia). To all the wells, 0.3 ml of culture oil is added (Culture Oil, Cook IVF). The dish is placed in an incubator until utilization.

The oocytes are rapidly incubated for 30 seconds (not more) in the hyaluronidase, passing them rapidly in and out of a glass Pasteur pipette. This operation permits liberation from the cumulus cells. At this point, the oocytes, surrounded only by corona cells, are moved into one of the wells filled with culture medium. The corona cells are removed by passing through progressively smaller capillaries (170 micrometers and 140 micrometers, Flexipet, Cook IVF). During this procedure, the oocytes are moved into the other wells filled with culture medium to reach a complete wash from the hyaluronidase. We do not usually recommend using capillaries with a diameter smaller than 140 micrometers, so that the sliding of the first PB into the perivitelline space (PVS) is avoided. However, if satisfactory denudation is not obtained, a smaller diameter can be used (130 micrometers).

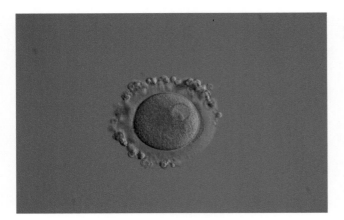

Figure 4.9 Very immature oocyte (prophase I) or germinal vesicle (GV).

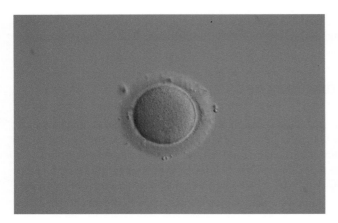

Figure 4.10 Immature oocyte (metaphase I). The first PB is absent.

After denudation, human oocyte consists of a cell (mean diameter of about 100–120 micrometers) surrounded by a trilaminar membrane (oolemma). External to the cell membrane, there is the ZP, which is separated from the oocyte by the PVS. The oocyte can show three different nuclear maturation stages:

1. Germinal vesicle (GV): the nucleus is clearly visible (Figure 4.9).
2. Metaphase I oocyte (MI): the nucleus has disappeared (GV breakdown) (Figure 4.10).
3. Metaphase II oocyte (MII): the first PB has been extruded in the PVS (Figure 4.11). It represents the end of nuclear oocyte maturation.

Evaluation of the cytoplasm

Cytoplasmic abnormalities

Cytoplasmic abnormalities are considered to be the most important feature in influencing the development potential. The cytoplasm can appear dark and granular. The granularity can be distributed homogenously or can be located in the middle and have different intensity. The central granularity is formed by organelle clusters and it can range from

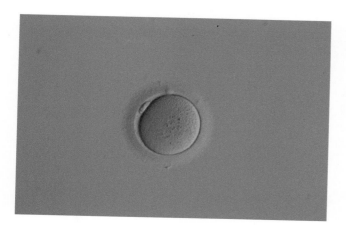

Figure 4.11 Mature oocyte (metaphase II). Note the presence of the first PB.

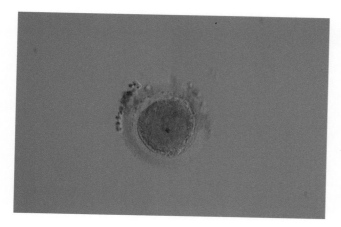

Figure 4.12 Degenerated oocyte. Note the irregular shape and dark cytoplasm.

light to severe. The evaluation of it is based on its diameter and depth (Kahraman *et al.*, 2000; Meriano *et al.*, 2001). In the cytoplasm we can observe oval, elliptical, smooth and flat formations which are formed by endoplasmic reticulum. We can often find one or more round cavities (vacuoles), "refractile body," which represent the inclusion of dark and necrotic material (Meriano *et al.*, 2001). It is possible to find oocytes with a large diameter from 30% to 200% of the norm. They are called "giant oocytes" and are commonly rejected because their chromosomes are very frequently abnormal (Funaki and Mikano, 1980; Balakier *et al.*, 2002). In addition to this, it is possible to find oocytes with reduced cytoplasm. Figures 4.12–4.20 show the most frequent ooplasmic abnormalities.

Extracytoplasmic abnormalities

These abnormalities also seem to be associated with oocyte function and development.

Zona pellucida (ZP) This can differ from the norm in its shape, color (dark) and thickness, which can be increased or decreased. Recent studies have pointed out that the

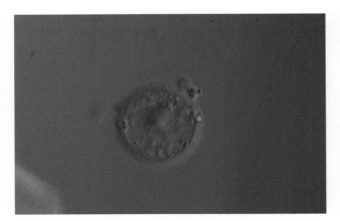

Figure 4.13 Empty zona: the ooplasm is absent.

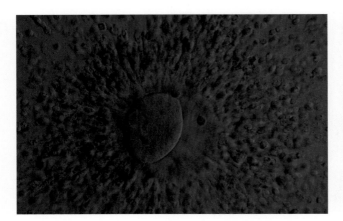

Figure 4.14 Oocyte with halved ooplasm.

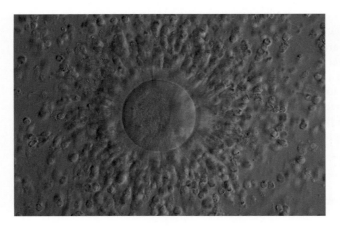

Figure 4.15 Mature oocyte surrounded by cumulus/corona cells. Note the severe central granulation of the ooplasm.

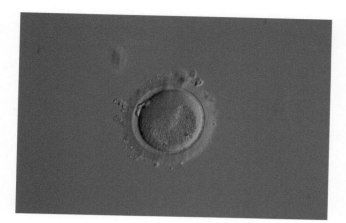

Figure 4.16 Denuded oocyte with severe ooplasm granulation that is moon shaped.

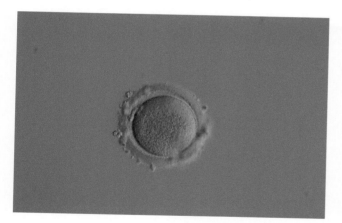

Figure 4.17 Denuded oocyte with granular ooplasm.

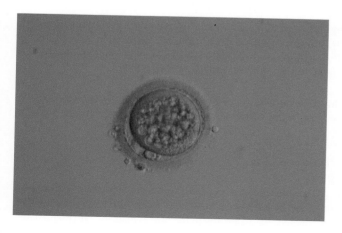

Figure 4.18 Oocyte with vacuolated ooplasm.

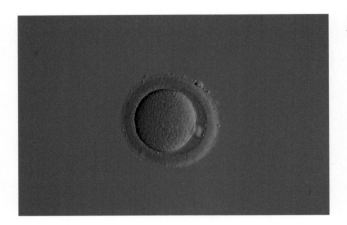

Figure 4.19 Mature oocyte with a cytoplasmic flat disk.

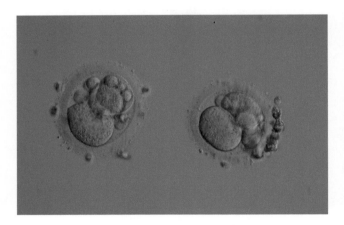

Figure 4.20 Oocytes with fragmented cytoplasm.

thickness of the ZP can change between different oocytes, although they belong to the same cohort (Pellettier *et al.*, 2004). Moreover, separations in the trilaminar structure can occur and form septa inside the PVS (Meriano *et al.*, 2001); structures on the external surface (brush-shape) that are similar to villi can also be observed.

Perivitelline space (PVS)   This can be absent when the oocyte has degenerated due to plasmatic membrane rupture, but, more often, it is too large because of the decrease in oocyte ooplasmic volume.

Perivitelline space granules   These appear as large dark granulations distributed around the oocyte in different concentrations.

First polar body fragmentation   The first PB may be of first or second grade (intact PB), and of third or fourth grade (fragmented PB) according to the post-ovulatory age (Eichenlaub-Ritter *et al.*, 1995; Ebner *et al.*, 1999, 2000).

Figures 4.21–4.26 show the more frequent extracytoplasmic abnormalities.

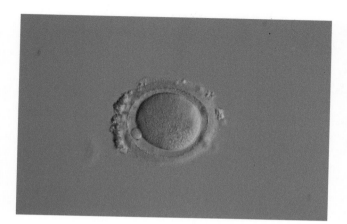

Figure 4.21 Oocyte with slightly increased perivitelline space (PVS).

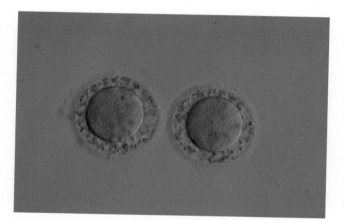

Figure 4.22 Oocytes with numerous PVS debris.

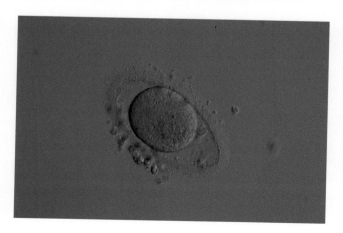

Figure 4.23 Oocyte with increased PVS and abnormal ZP.

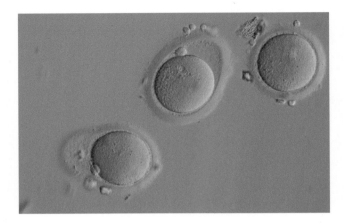

Figure 4.24 Oocytes with abnormal ZP shapes.

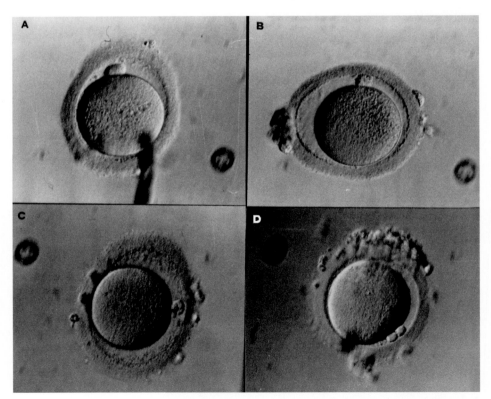

Figure 4.25 First PB classification. A: first grade; B: second grade; C: third grade; D: fourth grade. Produced from Ciotti *et al.* (2004).

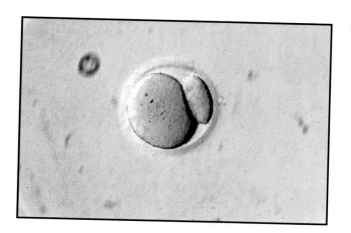

Figure 4.26 Giant first PB.

Evaluation of the meiotic spindle

Meiotic spindle can be evaluated by means of the PolScope. This instrument employs a technology studied by Oldenbourg (1996) and consists of a traditional polarized microscope which illuminates the sample with a circular polarizing light; the standard compensator is replaced by a liquid crystal-based one (LC) (liquid crystal-based orientation-independent polarizing light technology). The LC compensator and a CCD chamber are controlled by a computer. The LC compensator is set up in four different positions generating four images which are used to calculate the sample birefringence in all the pixels by using a patent polarimetric algorithm.

The data regarding the birefringence are kept in pixels and they are expressed through two different parameters: the amount of birefringence delay and the direction of the birefringence slow axis. In contrast to the images obtained through a conventional polarized microscope, the contrast of a birefringence structure in the image does not depend on the orientation of the sample.

This instrument permits the creation of an archive of the images to enable successive analyses. It is possible to measure length, angles and retardance. These parameters can be useful in carrying out evaluations on meiotic spindle quality and its repolymerization after thawing. The meiotic spindle is mostly constituted of proteins, so it tends to depolymerize at a non-physiological temperature and to repolymerize when the temperature is restored. The PolScope permits evaluation of this phenomenon by measuring the time for spindle recovery and its retardance.

For PolScope evaluation (LC-PolScope CRI Inc., Woburn, MA), a glass-bottomed culture dish (Will-Co-Well, Amsterdam, the Netherlands) with drops of 5 μl of culture medium covered by oil is prepared for each patient. A drop for each oocyte is prepared and another drop is used for instrument background. The PolScope must have a heated plate set at a temperature of 37 °C. A holding pipette is necessary in order to rotate the oocyte and to improve the possibility of visualization of the meiotic spindle during the observation. The PolScope is switched on and calibrated. The oocytes are placed one by one into the drops and the dish is put onto the microscope stage. After correcting the image for background, observation can start. Each oocyte is rotated with the help of the holding pipette until the meiotic spindle is viewable. If, after careful observation of the oocyte, the meiotic spindle is

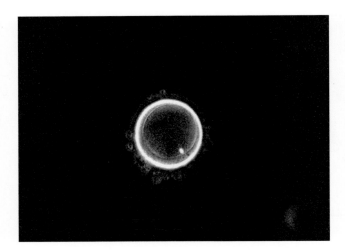

Figure 4.27 PolScope image of a metaphase II oocyte. Note the meiotic spindle aligned with the first PB.

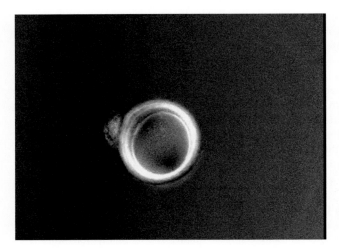

Figure 4.28 PolScope image of a metaphase II oocyte. The meiotic spindle is absent.

not viewable, the absence of the spindle will be registered. Figures 4.27–4.30 show some oocytes observed by PolScope to visualize the meiotic spindle.

Grading of the oocyte
The freezable egg score

A computerized egg score is based on several evaluations. The first evaluation is done by the stereomicroscope at egg retrieval. On the basis of the CCOC characteristics, the oocytes may be classified under the following categories: very immature, immature, mature and post-mature.

After denudation of the oocytes, the second evaluation may be done. The nuclear maturity is evaluated with the inverted microscope (20X) and the oocytes are grouped in the following categories: GV, metaphase I (no PB), metaphase II (first PB), degenerate, empty zone.

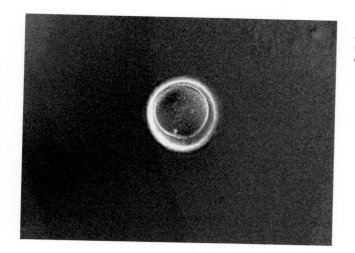

Figure 4.29 PolScope image of a metaphase II oocyte with the meiotic spindle slightly out of alignment from the first PB.

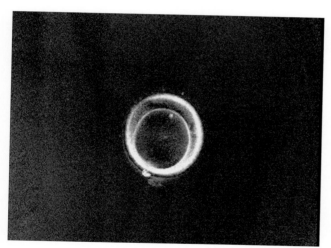

Figure 4.30 PolScope image of a metaphase II oocyte with the meiotic spindle strongly out of alignment from the first PB.

The mature oocytes (metaphase II) are further defined according to the cytoplasmic and extracytoplasmic abnormalities. Each characteristic is graded (Table 4.1). When several abnormalities are found in the same oocyte, the computer calculates the total score. Oocytes having a score ≤ 6 are considered suitable for cryopreservation. Oocytes with a higher score have a worse prognosis. The score will be evaluated again after thawing.

Survived oocyte

An oocyte which has truly survived after cryopreservation must appear morphologically as a fresh oocyte at the end of the thawing procedure. The definition of survival does not include the capacity to be fertilized. However, if the subsequent fertilization rate is strongly impaired, a more accurate assessment of the survival is advised.

Table 4.1. Score of normal/abnormal egg features

CHARACTERISTIC	SCORE
Perfect	0
Slight cytoplasmic granulation	1
Cytoplasmic granulation	4
Severe cytoplasmic granulation	8
Severe central granulation	9
Dark cytoplasm	7
Presence of cytoplasmic flat disk	7
Refractile body	1
Rare and small vacuoles	2
Wide and numerous vacuoles	8
Giant oocyte	9
Oocyte with abnormal shape (oval, etc.)	6
Oolemma breaking	9
Fragmented 1° PB	1
Degenerated 1° PB	3
Giant 1° PB	8
Abnormal ZP	6
ZP breaking	8
Increased PVS	7
Absent PVS	6
Rare PVS debris	1
Numerous PVS debris	7

Degenerated first polar body

It is not uncommon to find that an oocyte has survived with the first PB degenerated at the end of procedure. This oocyte can be used for insemination. It is important to register this finding to make a correct interpretation of subsequent fertilization. Figure 4.31 shows a survived oocyte with the first PB degenerated after thawing.

Degenerated oocyte

The cytoplasm is dark or transparent, the PVS is absent because of the oolemma rupture. The oocyte has to be discarded.

Oocyte with some sign of degeneration

The ooplasm is slightly dark and the PVS is reduced. This oocyte can be inseminated. However, the oocyte will be perceived to be less firm while injecting the sperm into the

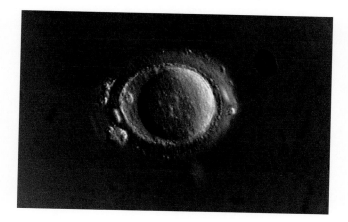

Figure 4.31 Metaphase II thawed oocyte. The oocyte survived but the first PB degenerated after thawing.

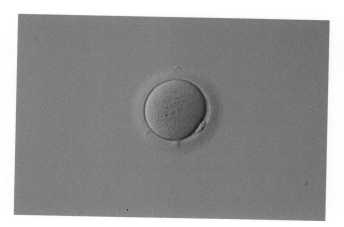

Figure 4.32 Metaphase II thawed oocyte. The oocyte survived. Note the homogeneous cytoplasm with a good rehydration and a regular PVS. This oocyte is suitable for ICSI.

cytoplasm. Although these oocytes can survive and be fertilized, they often degenerate immediately after intracytoplasmic sperm injection (ICSI) or later. In the last case, degeneration will be observed at the fertilization check.

In summary, oocyte degeneration may occur at thawing (during or at the end of the procedure) or after ICSI.

Figures 4.32–4.41 show a series of thawed oocytes with increasing and different post-thawing effects.

Steps and timing of the entire cryopreservation procedure
Timing of the events that occur after HCG administration until embryo transfer

HCG is administrated 36 hours before oocyte pickup. This timing is used to establish oocyte age. After at least 2 hours from pickup (38 hours after HCG), the oocytes can be denuded and the nuclear maturity can be evaluated. It is opportune to freeze the oocytes within 4–5 hours from retrieval (38–39 hours from HCG administration).

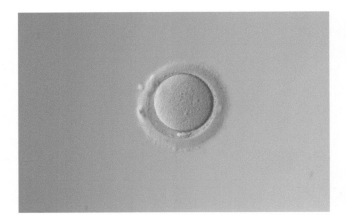

Figure 4.33 Metaphase II thawed oocyte. The oocyte survived. However, the cytoplasm is slightly granular. This oocyte is suitable for ICSI.

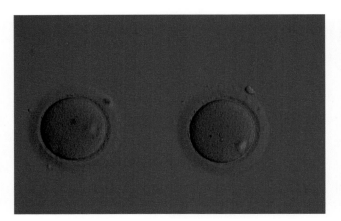

Figure 4.34 Two metaphase II thawed oocytes. The oocytes survived. Note the slightly granular cytoplasm. However, these oocytes are suitable for ICSI.

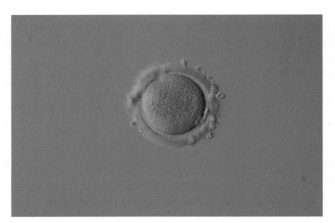

Figure 4.35 Metaphase II thawed oocyte. The oocyte survived but the cytoplasm is highly granular. However, this oocyte is suitable for ICSI.

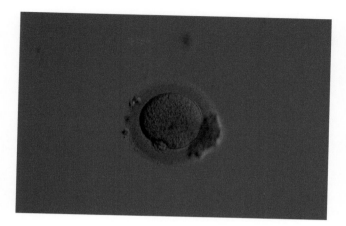

Figure 4.36 Metaphase II thawed oocyte. Note the highly granular and microvacuolated cytoplasm. It is not advised to utilize this oocyte for ICSI if other oocytes are available.

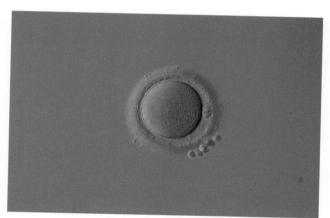

Figure 4.37 Metaphase II thawed oocyte. The cytoplasm rehydration is correct but the PVS is large. This oocyte is suitable for ICSI.

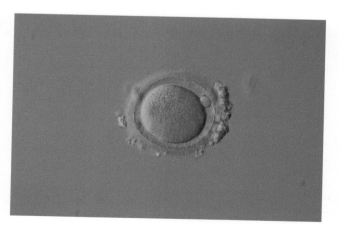

Figure 4.38 Metaphase II thawed oocyte. The cytoplasm rehydration is poor; however, the oocyte is suitable for ICSI.

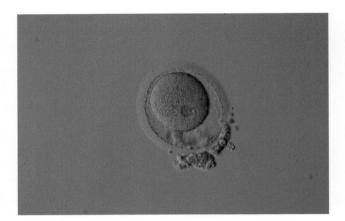

Figure 4.39 Metaphase II thawed oocyte. The cytoplasm displays a vacuole and poor rehydration. Note the very large PVS. It is advisable to discard this oocyte.

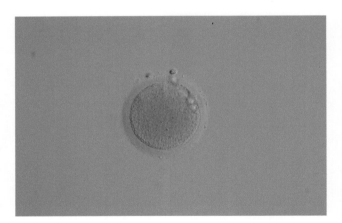

Figure 4.40 Metaphase II thawed oocyte. Note the dark cytoplasm and the absence of PVS. The oocyte is degenerated.

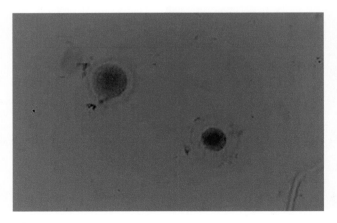

Figure 4.41 Metaphase II thawed oocytes. These oocytes degenerated as demonstrated by the trypan blue staining: the cell membrane lost its selective permeability and the trypan blue dyes the cytoplasm by osmosis.

The end of the thawing procedure, when the oocytes are put into culture, is considered to be "time 0." Insemination must occur within 2–3 hours from time 0 in order to have a total culture time not exceeding 6–7 hours. According to recent data regarding the spindle recovery after vitrification (Gardner *et al.*, 2007; Larman *et al.*, 2007b; Ciotti *et al.*, 2009), the time of culture after warming could be decreased to one hour so that the damages related to in vitro aging are reduced.

Fertilization is checked within 18 hours after the insemination, as is the case for fresh oocytes. The embryo check is carried out on the second to third day. It is important to point out that cleavage of these embryos is slightly lower when compared with that of fresh embryos; thus, four-cell embryos are frequently found on the third day.

Timing of semen sample production

The biologist does not proceed to thaw the oocytes until the presence of sperms in the sample is confirmed. If the semen has been cryopreserved, the biologist does not proceed to oocyte thawing until he is sure that sperms have been found in the sample.

Organizing criteria for storage in liquid nitrogen tanks

The subdivision of the oocytes in the storing devices (straws or others) at the moment of freezing is determined by oocyte maturity, the presence/absence of the meiotic spindle and patient age. At the moment of thawing, the aim is to not waste oocytes and to obtain three oocytes capable of being inseminated. It means that we try to obtain the number of oocytes that we decided to inseminate without the risk to obtain supernumerary embryos.

Cryobiology

Cryobiology is the scientific study of the effects of low temperatures on living systems. Knowledge and understanding of the main principles of cryobiology are fundamental. In order to get good results you must rigorously apply theoretical considerations and empirical observations derived from studies on different types of cells. Cryopreservation foresees that biological material is brought to temperatures at which chemical, biological and physical activity is suspended. It is very complex to establish procedures which bring biological samples from a physiological temperature ($37\,^\circ$C) to a cryogenic temperature ($-196\,^\circ$C) while maintaining high percentages of survival. The factors playing a fundamental role in cryopreservation are morphological (dimensions, maturity, quality of the cell) and biophysical (cryoprotectants, speed of freezing and thawing).

The phase of transition from water to ice is very important because of the abundance of water inside the cells. At temperatures below $-0.6\,^\circ$C, biological water becomes thermodynamically unstable and transformation to the crystalline state is facilitated. Therefore, the speed of freezing-thawing becomes extremely important because it establishes the final destiny of intracellular water.

Water is a universal solvent. It has bipolar characteristics which allow it to participate in multiple hydrogen bonds, which stabilize important biological structures. The phase of transition, during the formation of ice, destroys these properties and is one of the principal causes of "cryopreservation damage." Modern cryobiology is based on the discovery that there are other solutes which can replace some of the properties of water, developing a cryoprotective action. These mechanisms represent one of the evolutionary strategies employed by many animals and implantations which succeed in surviving at freezing temperatures in extreme environments. Cryoprotectants belong to two broad categories according to their molecular weight: those permeating the membrane and those not permeating the membrane. The former (glycerol, DMSO [dimethyl sulfoxide], ethylene glycol [EG], 1,2-propanediol [PROH]) can cross the cellular membrane with different characteristics of permeability, replacing some of the functions of the water; they lower the freezing point and protect the membranes from possible ultrastructural modifications which can occur during cooling. However, they can become toxic with an increase in concentration, temperature and time of exposure. The non-permeating cryoprotectants (sucrose, threalose, Ficoll, polyvinylpyrrolidone [PVP]) cannot cross the cellular membrane and their mechanism of action is based on the creation of an osmotic gradient which helps the dehydration of the cell. They are usually used in association with permeating cryoprotectants. Their function of substituting water, which is so important at low temperatures, also means that they possess an innate toxicity if they are used on cells at physiological temperatures. Toxicity is proportional to the concentration and the time of exposure. A correct compromise must be sought for each type of cell.

Cryoprotectants are added and removed in a gradual way in order to reduce the excessive osmotic gradients which can arise. It is also necessary to balance the benefits of the slow addition of the cryoprotectants with the deleterious effects caused by the consequent increase in the time of exposure.

The formation of intracellular ice is the principal cause of cryopreservation damage. Its formation is influenced by the surface/volume relationship of the cell, by the characteristics of the permeability of the cell and by the speed of freezing. For each type of cell, a specific curve of cooling showing optimal survival must be identified.

The consequent cryodamage can affect every part of the oocyte:

Extracytoplasmatic damage: degeneration of the first PB, breakage and hardening of the ZP.

Cytoplasmatic damage: breakage of the oolemma; degeneration of the ooplasm; the loss of mitochondria with a consequent loss of energy; the loss of cortical granules with the consequent problems of fertilization (polyspermy) and damage to the cytoskeleton, to the chromosome and to the meiotic spindle with consequent possible aneuploidy.

Chapter 5

Slow freezing

Principles

Slow freezing requires the use of cryoprotectants and a slow decrease of the temperature. During the passage from $-5\,^{\circ}C$ to $-15\,^{\circ}C$, the cell progressively loses water by osmosis and the formation of extracellular ice occurs. This causes an increase in the concentration of solutes in the extracellular environment with the consequent increase in the osmotic gradient and additional cellular dehydration. Cellular volume decreases and dehydration is progressive. The passage must be long enough to allow sufficient extraction of the water from the cell and to reduce the super cooling of the cytoplasm and keep the formation of intracellular ice crystals to a minimum. In nature, the formation of ice in a sufficiently cooled solution is casual and spontaneous. To overcome this problem, the formation of extracellular ice is induced by a process called "seeding." It consists of provoking the formation of the first extracellular crystal of ice in a precise point and at an established temperature. From this point, the extracellular ice increases, causing progressive cell dehydration.

During thawing, small particles of the intracellular ice which were formed during freezing can unite, forming a larger crystal (recrystallization). The mechanisms by which heating influences cell survival are not well known, but it seems that rapid heating is efficacious in reducing the formation of intracellular crystals during this phase and therefore in reducing damage. The cryoprotectants are removed step by step in order to avoid osmotic shock.

Evolution of the slow freezing methodology

The first studies on the cryopreservation of mouse oocytes were carried out by Whittingam et al. (1972) using dimethyl sulfoxide (DMSO) as a cryoprotectant, utilizing a curve of slow freezing set up for the embryos. The results were fair in terms of survival but not in terms of development and implantation. Poor results were also obtained with other animal species. The first results regarding the cryopreservation of human oocytes were obtained with DMSO and slow freezing with a varying survival rate of between 20% and 80% (Chen, 1986; Al-Hasani et al., 1987; van Uem et al., 1987; Mandelbaum 1988a, 1988b) and 0% (Trounson, 1986). However, in this period, the first pregnancies were obtained (Chen 1986; Van Uem et al., 1987). Subsequently, good results were achieved in terms of survival (60%) using 1,2-propanediol (PROH) as a cryoprotectant (Trounson, 1986). The studies of Renard and Babinot (1984) showed that PROH was less toxic than DMSO and other authors (Lassalle et al., 1985) stated that it was appropriate for the cryopreservation of mouse oocytes and human embryos. Some authors showed that exposure to PROH without cryopreservation did not have consequences on fertilization and embryonic development (Bernard *et al.*, 1985) while others did not find any improvement in comparison to DMSO (Mandelbaum *et al.*, 1988b), also when adding sucrose (Al-Hasani *et al.*, 1987; Mandelbaum *et al.*, 1988b).

In the years following these scarce results, oocyte cryopreservation did not arouse great interest. Hope was revived by studies in 1993 (Gook *et al.*, 1993) in which PROH and sucrose (0.1 M) were used, obtaining approximately 60% post-thawing survival. With the same method, Kazem *et al.* (1995) and Tucker *et al.* (1996) obtained lower percentages of survival (34% and 25%) and in 1997 (Porcu *et al.*, 1997), the first birth from cryopreserved oocytes was obtained with the use of ICSI as an insemination technique. Subsequently, the association of oocyte cryopreservation and ICSI has found wider use and numerous pregnancies have been obtained by various groups in different parts of the world (Antinori *et al.*, 1998; Borini *et al.*, 1998, 2004, 2006a; Porcu *et al.*, 1998, 1999b, 2000a, 2001, 2002, 2008). These results were obtained by using (without modifications) the method of cryo-preservation for embryos developed by Lassalle *et al.* (1985). The introduction of ICSI has surely offered great advantages, providing the possibility of obtaining a greater number of fertilized oocytes and, therefore, of transferable embryos.

Subsequently, the study of the factors which could influence the survival of oocytes after thawing was initiated. An increase in the concentration of sucrose from 0.1 M to 0.2 M and 0.3 M (Fabbri *et al.*, 2001) with a consequent increase in cell dehydration has offered the possibility of improving survival to approximately 80%. Higher concentrations of sucrose (0.2 M, 0.3 M) have subsequently been used by many groups, maintaining survival at approximately 70%. However, clinical results have not been as satisfactory. A large-scale review of the cryopreservation of human oocytes includes a summary of the rates of implantation obtained with the various protocols (Gook and Edgar, 2007): 1.5 M PROH + 0.1 M sucrose = 10%; 1.5 M PROH + 0.2 M sucrose = 17%; 1.5 M PROH + 0.3 M sucrose = 5%. From these results it seems that the use of 0.3 M sucrose results in higher survival and, therefore, a greater number of oocytes capable of being fertilized, but it also seems that developed embryos have a smaller probability of implantation. It must be considered that, in this review, the results with 0.2 M sucrose include both results obtained with 0.2 M sucrose in solutions of freezing and thawing, and those achieved with diversified concentrations: 0.2 M sucrose in freezing and 0.3 M sucrose in thawing (Bianchi *et al.*, 2007). Bianchi *et al.* (2007) utilized a modified version of the conventional slow freezing protocol: 0.2 M sucrose was used in the freezing phase to assure sufficient dehydration and a more elevated concentration (0.3 M) of sucrose was used in the rehydration phase to achieve more controlled rehydration. These first results, obtained on 403 thawed oocytes, showed survival of 75.9%, a rate of fertilization of 76.2% and 86.2% of good quality embryos. The rate of implantation was 13.5%.

A study was carried out with confocal microscopy to examine the effect of the concentration of sucrose (0.1 M or 0.3 M) on the meiotic spindle and chromosomal configuration after slow freezing (Coticchio *et al.*, 2006). The data show that the protocol having a more elevated concentration of sucrose promotes the maintenance of a normal apparatus for chromosomal segregation similar to that which is found in fresh oocytes. A study (Nottola *et al.*, 2007) on the ultrastructure of cryopreserved human oocytes using different concentrations of sucrose (0.1 M or 0.3 M) in the freezing solution, shows that the organelles are numerous and uniformly distributed in the ooplasm, the quantity of cortical granules is lower in frozen-thawed oocytes independent of the concentration of sucrose utilized, and that a slightly higher microvacuolization occurs in the ooplasm of oocytes frozen in 0.3 M sucrose. Vacuolization has a negative prognostic effect on embryonic development.

Recently, the use of increasing concentrations of ethylene glycol (EG) and 0.2 M sucrose as cryoprotectants has been investigated experimentally on mature human oocytes. The results do not favor the use of EG because ultrastructural analysis shows various alterations, among which some delamination of the zona pellucida and ooplasmic vacuolization (Nottola *et al.*, 2008).

Another change applied to slow freezing is the use of sodium-free, phosphate-buffered saline (PBS) as a base for the preparation of cryopreservation solutions. A study carried out on mouse oocytes has ascertained that sodium is the most abundant salt of cryopreservation solutions and is, therefore, the principal agent responsible for the so-called "solution effects," which, together with the formation of intracellular ice, represent the most deleterious events for the cryopreservation of cells (Stachecki *et al.*, 1998). In place of the sodium, choline is used as the most concentrated extracellular cation. Choline does not cross the cellular membrane and therefore it does not contribute to the concentration of intracellular ions, which, if excessively elevated, is incompatible with normal cellular functions. The cryopreservation solutions that are based on sodium-free PBS are called "depleted PBS solution" because there is a quantity of sodium present in the serum component that is always added to cryopreservation solutions. Depleted PBS freezing solutions with different concentrations of sucrose have been used, from a clinical point of view, by different authors. Gook and Edgar (2007) showed a cumulative implantation rate of 21%, 11% and 16% utilizing 0.1 M sucrose, 0.2 M sucrose and 0.3 M sucrose, respectively. The data referred to samples of rather reduced entity. In the study of Stachecki *et al.* (1998), the problem of the presence of a protein component in the freezing solutions was addressed. In this study on mouse oocytes, an increase in the concentration of bovine serum improved the rate of fertilization and development due to the protective effect that the protein component has on the membranes.

A large study pointed out the importance of the physiological characteristics of the female gametes in obtaining satisfactory results in cryopreservation (Gardner *et al.*, 2007). It was observed that exposure to any permeating cryoprotectants provokes an increase in the intracellular concentration of calcium similar to that instigated by the entrance of the sperm during fertilization with a consequent phenomenon of zona hardening. Larman *et al.* (2007a), by studying the effect of PROH on mouse oocytes, reported that this cryoprotectant induces the entrance of enough extracellular calcium to cause zona hardening, and they therefore recommend the use of calcium-deprived solutions to reduce this phenomenon. Ethylene glycol, in comparison to PROH and DMSO, is the cryoprotectant which causes the smallest and briefest peak of calcium on mouse oocytes. The elimination of calcium from freezing solutions notably reduces the effect of PROH and EG while DMSO is not influenced by it, showing that the first two cryoprotectants exert their effects by acting on the entrance of extracellular calcium while the third one has a direct action on the mitochondria and the endoplasmic reticulum. The data obtained on mouse oocytes suggest that the use of DMSO is not advisable for their cryopreservation and that the concentration of calcium should be evaluated in the freezing solutions in which PROH and EG are used (Gardner *et al.*, 2007).

Slow freezing/rapid thawing

The preparation of all solutions, and the procedures, has to be done under laminar flow and reduced artificial light conditions.

Materials

REAGENTS FOR SOLUTIONS	
PBS = Phosphate buffered saline	GIBCO INVITROGEN, NY, USA
DSS = Dextran serum supplement	Irvine Scientific, Santa Ana, California
PROH = 1,2-propanediol	Fluka Chemika, Sigma–Aldrich, the Netherlands
SUCROSE extra pure, m. wt. = 342,3	Sigma–Aldrich, the Netherlands

TOOLS FOR SLOW FREEZING	
STRAW Crystal	Cryo Bio System, IMV Technologies, France
INSULIN TYPE SYRINGE 1 ml	
MILLEX-GP 0.22 µm Filter Unit	MILLIPORE (Millipore, Bedford, MA)
SILICONE TUBE inner diameter 1.5 mm, outer diameter 3.5 mm	
JONC	Cryo Bio System, IMV Technologies, France
GOBLET diameter 12 mm	Cryo Bio System, IMV Technologies, France
GOBLET diameter 65 mm	Cryo Bio System, IMV Technologies, France
METAL STICK	Cryo Bio System, IMV Technologies, France
TIMER	

TOOLS FOR THAWING	
WATER-BATH 30 °C	
THERMOMETER	
STERILE SCISSORS	

DISPOSABLE MATERIALS	
FLASK 50 ml	Falcon, Becton Dickinson, NJ, USA
PETRI DISH 35 x 10 mm	Falcon, Becton Dickinson, NJ, USA
TUBE 13 ml	Falcon, Becton Dickinson, NJ, USA
SEROLOGICAL PIPETTE 10 ml	Falcon, Becton Dickinson, NJ, USA

(cont.)

DISPOSABLE MATERIALS

SEROLOGICAL PIPETTE 1 ml	Falcon, Becton Dickinson, NJ, USA
MULTIDISH 4 WELLS Nunclon	NUNC, Denmark
PRE-STERILIZED/PRE-PLUGGED PASTEUR PIPETTE	Poulten-Graf Ltd., England
STERILE SYRINGE 10 ml	
SURGICAL GAUZE	

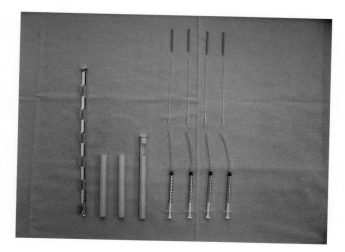

Figure 5.1 Materials necessary for slow freezing. From the left: one metal stick to keep the goblet (it must be marked in the upper part); three green goblets to contain the straws (the third goblet is already joined to the metal stick); four insulin type syringes with a small silicone tube that will join the syringe to the straw during the sample loading; four straws supplied with a yellow jonc that has already been identified with the surname, name and number of samples.

Figure 5.1 illustrates the materials necessary for slow freezing. From the left:

- Metal stick. The upper portion must be labeled and its function is to hold the goblet
- Two green goblets are used to contain the straws, the third one is already attached to the metal stick
- Four insulin type syringes are connected with a small silicone tube. They are used to join the syringe to the straw during the sample loading
- Straws. They are supplied with a yellow jonc that has already been identified with the surname, name and number of samples.

Solutions for slow freezing

Detailed recipes of the freezing protocols are listed:

- PROH – 0.1 M sucrose
- PROH – 0.2 M sucrose
- PROH – 0.3 M sucrose
- PROH and differential sucrose concentrations
- PBS – Na^+ depleted.

Freezing solutions for human oocytes are 1.5 M PROH, 0.1 M sucrose:

There are three freezing solutions (FS). FS1 is a wash solution, FS2 is the first dehydration solution, and FS3 is the second dehydration solution and is also the solution in which the samples are loaded into the straw.

Prepare the solutions in Falcon Tube 13 ml.

SOLUTION	COMPOSITION/PREPARATION	FILTRATION
FREEZING SOLUTION 1 **(Wash solution)**	**PBS + 30% DSS** 7 ml PBS + 3 ml DSS	Filter into a new Falcon Tube 13 ml
FREEZING SOLUTION 2 **(Dehydration solution)**	**1.5 M PROH + 30% DSS** 5.86 ml PBS + 1.14 ml PROH + 3 ml DSS	Filter into a new Falcon Tube 13 ml
FREEZING SOLUTION 3 **(Dehydration and loading solution)**	**1.5 M PROH + 0.1 M SUCROSE + 30% DSS** 0.342 g SUCROSE + 4 ml PBS + 1.14 ml PROH and solubilize; make up to a volume of 7 ml with PBS. Add 3 ml DSS	Filter into a new Falcon Tube 13 ml

Thawing solutions for human oocytes

There are four thawing solutions. The cryoprotectant concentrations decrease from the first until the fourth solution to obtain the slow rehydration of the samples.

Prepare the mother solutions in a 50 ml flask and the final solutions in Falcon Tube 13 ml.

SOLUTION	COMPOSITION/PREPARATION
MOTHER SOLUTION 1	**1.0 M PROH** 14.78 ml PBS + 1.217 ml PROH
MOTHER SOLUTION 2	**0.5 M PROH** 4 ml PBS + 4 ml mother solution 1

SOLUTION	COMPOSITION/PREPARATION	FILTRATION
THAWING SOLUTION 1	**1.0 M PROH + 0.1 M SUCROSE + 30% DSS** 0.342 g SUCROSE + 5 ml mother solution 1 and solubilize; make up to a volume of 7 ml with mother solution 1. Add 3 ml DSS	Filter into a new Falcon Tube 13 ml
THAWING SOLUTION 2	**0.5 M PROH + 0.1 M SUCROSE + 30% DSS** 0.342 g SUCROSE + 5 ml mother solution 2 and solubilize; make up to a volume of 7 ml with mother solution 2. Add 3 ml DSS	Filter into a new Falcon Tube 13 ml

(cont.)

SOLUTION	COMPOSITION/PREPARATION	FILTRATION
THAWING SOLUTION 3	**0.1 M SUCROSE + 30% DSS** 0.342 g SUCROSE + 5 ml PBS and solubilize; make up to a volume of 7 ml with PBS. Add 3 ml DSS	Filter into a new Falcon Tube 13 ml
THAWING SOLUTION 4	**PBS + 30% DSS** 7 ml PBS Add 3 ml DSS	Filter into a new Falcon Tube 13 ml

Freezing and thawing solutions have to be filtered starting from the least to higher concentrated ones. They have to be stored at +4 °C.

The solutions can be stored and utilized for 60 days from the day of preparation if they are stored correctly. The date of preparation is utilized as LOT Number. They are listed in an informatized inventory.

To obtain the solutions at 0.2 M sucrose and 0.3 M sucrose it is necessary to multiply by 2 and by 3 the sucrose concentration indicated in the previous recipe for 0.1 M sucrose.

Setting up for a freezing cycle

Set up one 4 wells Nunclon for each straw.

POSITION	SOLUTION and VOLUME
1° WELL	1° FREEZING SOL. (WASH SOL) 0.5 ml
2° WELL	2° FREEZING SOL. (DEHYDRATION SOL) 0.5 ml
3° WELL	3° FREEZING SOL. (LOADING SOL) 0.5 ml

Setting up for a thawing cycle

Set up one 4 wells Nunclon for each straw.

POSITION	SOLUTION and VOLUME
1° WELL	1° THAWING SOL. 0.5 ml
2° WELL	2° THAWING SOL. 0.5 ml
3° WELL	3° THAWING SOL. 0.5 ml
4° WELL	4° THAWING SOL. 0.5 ml

Freezing solutions at different sucrose concentrations

(0.2 M during freezing, 0.3 M during thawing.)

There are three freezing solutions (FS). FS1 and FS2 are dehydration solutions, FS3 is the third dehydration solution and it is also the solution in which the samples are loaded into the straw.

Prepare the solutions in Falcon Tube 13 ml.

SOLUTION	COMPOSITION/PREPARATION	FILTRATION
FREEZING SOLUTION 1 **(Dehydration solution)**	**0.75 M PROH + 20% DSS** 7.43 ml PBS + 0.57 PROH + 2 ml DSS	Filter into a new Falcon Tube 13 ml
FREEZING SOLUTION 2 **(Dehydration solution)**	**1.5 M PROH + 20% DSS** 6.86 ml PBS + 1.14 ml PROH + 2 ml DSS	Filter into a new Falcon Tube 13 ml
FREEZING SOLUTION 3 **(Dehydration and loading solution)**	**1.5 M PROH + 0.2 M SUCROSE + 20% DSS** 0.684 g SUCROSE + 4 ml PBS + 1.14 ml PROH and solubilize; make up to a volume of 8ml with PBS. Add 2 ml DSS	Filter into a new Falcon Tube 13 ml

Store at +4 °C.

Thawing solutions with differentiated sucrose concentrations

(0.2 M for freezing solutions, 0.3 M for thawing solutions.)

There are four thawing solutions. The cryoprotectant concentrations decrease from the first through the fourth solution to obtain the slow rehydration of the samples.

Prepare the mother solutions in a 50 ml flask and the final solutions in Falcon Tube 13 ml.

SOLUTION	COMPOSITION/PREPARATION
MOTHER SOLUTION 1	**1.0 M PROH** 14.78 ml PBS + 1.217 ml PROH
MOTHER SOLUTION 2	**0.5 M PROH** 4 ml PBS + 4 ml of mother solution 1

SOLUTION	COMPOSITION/PREPARATION	FILTRATION
THAWING SOLUTION 1	**1.0 M PROH + 0.3 M SUCROSE + 20% DSS** 1.026 g SUCROSE + 5 ml mother solution 1 and solubilize; make up to a volume of 8ml with mother solution 1. Add 2 ml DSS	Filter into a new Falcon Tube 13 ml
THAWING SOLUTION 2	**0.5 M PROH + 0.3 M SUCROSE + 20% SSS** 1.026 g SUCROSE + 5 ml mother solution 2 and solubilize; make up to a volume of 8 ml with mother solution 2. Add 2 ml DSS	Filter into a new Falcon Tube 13 ml
THAWING SOLUTION 3	**0.3 M SUCROSE + 20% DSS** 1.026 g SUCROSE + 5 ml PBS and solubilize; make up to a volume of 8 ml with PBS. Add 2 ml DSS	Filter into a new Falcon Tube 13 ml

(*cont.*)

SOLUTION	COMPOSITION/PREPARATION	FILTRATION
THAWING SOLUTION 4	**PBS + 20% DSS** 8 ml PBS Add 2 ml DSS	Filter into a new Falcon Tube 13 ml

Store at +4 °C.

Freezing and thawing solutions have to be filtered starting from the least to higher concentrated ones. They have to be stored at +4 °C.

The solutions can be stored and utilized for 60 days from the day of preparation if they are stored correctly. The day of preparation is utilized as LOT Number.

Setting up for a freezing cycle with differential sucrose concentrations

Set up one 4 wells Nunclon for each straw.

POSITION	SOLUTION and VOLUME
1° WELL	1° FREEZING SOL. (DEHYDRATION SOL) 0.5 ml
2° WELL	2° FREEZING SOL. (DEHYDRATION SOL) 0.5 ml
3° WELL	3° FREEZING SOL. (DEHYDRATION and LOADING SOL) 0.5 ml

Setting up for a thawing cycle with differential sucrose concentrations

Set up one 4 wells Nunclon for each straw.

POSITION	SOLUTION and VOLUME
1° WELL	1° THAWING SOL. 0.5 ml
2° WELL	2° THAWING SOL. 0.5 ml
3° WELL	3° THAWING SOL. 0.5 ml
4° WELL	4° THAWING SOL. 0.5 ml

Recipe formula for Na depleted PBS

COMPONENT	QUANTITY
Potassium chloride	99 mg (Sigma–Aldrich)
Disodium phosphate dodecahydrate	1.44 g (Sigma–Aldrich)

(cont.)

COMPONENT	QUANTITY
Monobasic potassium phosphate	100 mg (Sigma–Aldrich)
Choline chloride	9.55 g (Sigma–Aldrich)
Water for embryo transfer	500 ml (Sigma–Aldrich)

The PBS solutions obtained in this way will be used as the basis for the freezing and thawing solutions described above. Solutions will be supplemented with 20% DSS.

Volume, temperature and time of exposure during slow freezing utilizing solutions with 0.1 or 0.2 or 0.3 M sucrose at freezing and thawing (freezing 0.1 M/thawing 0.1 M–freezing 0.2 M/thawing 0.2 M–freezing 0.3 M/thawing 0.3 M)

Solutions with increasing cryoprotectant molarity.

SOLUTION	VOLUME	INCUBATION TIME	TEMPERATURE
Sol. 1 = wash sol. (PBS + 30% DSS)	0.5 ml	A brief wash	RT
Sol. 2 = dehydration sol. (1.5 M PROH + 30% DSS)	0.5 ml	10 min	RT
Sol. 3 = dehydration sol. (1.5 M PROH + 0.1 or 0.2 or 0.3 M sucrose + 30% DSS)	0.5 ml	10 min*	RT

* This time could be slightly different depending on the number of oocytes for freezing cycle.
RT = room temperature.

Volume, temperature and time of exposure during slow freezing utilizing solutions with differentiated sucrose concentrations (freezing 0.2 M sucrose/thawing 0.3 M)

Solutions with increasing cryoprotectant molarity.

SOLUTION	VOLUME	INCUBATION TIME	TEMPERATURE
Sol. 1 = dehydration sol. (0.75 M PROH + 20% DSS)	0.5 ml	7.5 min	RT
Sol. 2 = dehydration sol. (1.5 M PROH + 20% DSS)	0.5 ml	7.5 min	RT
Sol. 3 = dehydration and loading sol. (1.5 M PROH + 0.2 M sucrose + 20% DSS)	0.5 ml	5 min*	RT

* This time could be slightly different depending on the number of oocytes for the freezing cycle.
RT = room temperature.

Figure 5.2 shows the 4 wells Nunclon utilized during the samples' exposure to the cryoprotectants. Figure 5.3 illustrates the reduction of ooplasm volume during exposure to the cryoprotectants.

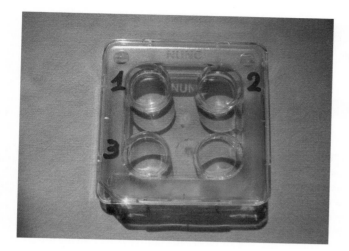

Figure 5.2 4 wells Nunclon utilized for slow freezing. The numbers identify the freezing solutions

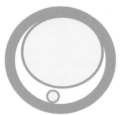

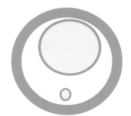

Figure 5.3 Reduction of the cytoplasmic volume during incubation in the cryoprotectants.

Time = 0 min

Time = 15 min
(−40% of the original volume)

Starting the freezing cycle

When all the material is ready, the programmable freezer is turned on and the timer is set; the oocytes are taken from the incubator and put under the laminar flow hood. They are taken and distributed in the well containing the first solution, as previously established. The countdown begins when the first oocytes are placed in incubation solution 1. When this first period has finished, the samples are moved to the following solution, beginning with the first oocytes which were incubated. The passages between one solution and another are carried out by collecting the oocytes in a small amount of the solution in which they are found and releasing them into the successive solution. This procedure makes the passage from one molarity to another less shocking.

When the passages are finished, the loading is carried out. The necessary number of straws has already been connected to the syringes and the colored joncs have already been labeled (surname, name and number of oocytes). Beginning with the first oocytes which were incubated, a straw is taken and the loading begins as shown in Figure 5.4. This step has a variable duration which depends on the number of oocytes to be frozen.

Each plug jonc must be firmly inserted into the loaded straw, checking that they correspond. This operation is carried out by a second person who assists the operator

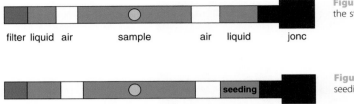

Figure 5.4 Modality of loading the straw for slow freezing

filter liquid air   sample   air   liquid   jonc

Figure 5.5 Correct position for seeding.

during the freezing process. The two operators check each other. Figure 5.4 illustrates the modality of loading the straw; it is the same for all the slow freezing solutions.

The straw is loaded as previously described by keeping the sample in the middle of the liquid and separating it from the margins by means of air bubbles. Another two small parts of the liquid isolate the sample at the filter side and at the plug side. It is important to try to place all the samples at approximately the same height so that there is simultaneous ice formation in all the samples (after seeding). The air blocks the sample from moving towards the external sides and the small quantity of liquid represents a safety measure at the moment of cutting the straw at thawing.

Loading the straw into the programmable freezer

After placing the labeling jonc, the straw is separated from the syringe which was used for loading and is inserted into the programmable freezer. At most, two straws are placed in each position. The position is closed through a safety device.

Beginning of the freezing program

When all the straws have been loaded, the operator gives the machine, which is at a starting temperature of $20\,^{\circ}\text{C}$, the command to RUN and the program begins.

Seeding

This is the induction of the first nucleus of ice into the extracellular solution. After approximately 20 minutes, the program provides a time of soaking at $-7\,^{\circ}\text{C}$. The program advises when it is the right moment for seeding with an acoustic and visual signal. The operator partially immerses metal forceps into the liquid nitrogen. The straws in one position are removed, rapidly but not completely, and the straws are tightened in the forceps in the indicated position (Figure 5.5). Immediately after forming the first ice nucleus, the straws are delicately released into position, which is then closed with the safety device. When the seeding has been done for all the straws, the RUN button to restart the program is pressed again. The seeding is manually induced by touching the part of the straw indicated with forceps cooled to $-196\,^{\circ}\text{C}$.

Storage of the samples

When the programmable freezer has reached a temperature of $-150\,^{\circ}\text{C}$, the program ends. The program provides for this temperature to be maintained for two hours so that the operator does not have to be present at the exact moment the program finishes. It is advisable to leave the samples at $-150\,^{\circ}\text{C}$ for at least 10 minutes to stabilize the temperature.

Meanwhile, the operator prepares the goblet (without making holes in the plastic) and the metal stick, labeled with the patient's name and surname. The operator plunges the goblet and the metal stick into a small container filled with liquid nitrogen and decides the positions of the samples for definitive storage. He/she removes the straws from each position and plunges them into the liquid nitrogen.

When all the straws of a patient are in the small container filled with liquid nitrogen, they are inserted into the goblet using forceps. The loaded goblet is picked up with forceps and positioned in the predetermined definitive position (dewar and canister).

The programmable freezer gives a signal when the program finishes advising that the samples can be removed. When all the straws have been removed from the instrument, the RUN key is pressed and the temperature begins to increase. The instrument must not be switched off until it has reached the starting temperature (20 °C). Now the programmable freezer could begin another freezing cycle. If this is not necessary, the instrument can be switched off and the safety valve of the pressure pump can be opened to reset it at zero. The safety valve is left open when the instrument is not in use.

Figure 5.6 illustrates the graphic of the freezing curve. The freezing curve is described in detail and, as concerns slow freezing, it is the same for the different freezing solutions.

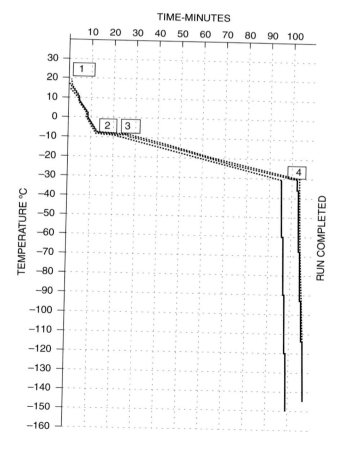

Figure 5.6 Graphic of the freezing curve.

STEP	FREEZING RATE
START: 20 °C	
1°	–2 °C/min until at –7 °C
2°	Hold –7 °C for 10 min. Seeding time after 3 min
3°	–0,3 °C/min until –30 °C
4°	–50 °C/min until –150 °C
5°	Hold –150 °C for 2 hours

Leave the samples for at least 10 minutes at −150 °C before taking them out from the machine for storing.

The total consumption of liquid nitrogen for a freezing cycle is about 10 liters.

Automated computerized freezing machine

This instrument has the capability of carrying out the programmed cooling of biological samples within temperatures ranging from +30 °C to −180 °C. The most commonly utilized is from Planer (Planer, Sunbury-On-Thames, United Kingdom). It is composed of a chamber which contains the samples and a programmable temperature control mechanism with an integrated display and an alphanumeric graph to register the data (Figure 4.2). It is connected to a liquid nitrogen dewar equipped with a pump, which feeds nitrogen to the chamber, and a control. The dewar is positioned on a portable platform. The chamber allows the freezing of different types of devices maintained in different positions.

The freezing is regulated through the controlled injection of atomized liquid nitrogen and through the ignition of a warmer which is activated by a programmable controller inside the chamber. This duplex action permits accurate cooling or warming inside the chamber. The chamber temperature is measured with a thermometer having a platinum resistance situated at the base of the chamber. It emits a signal which is transmitted to the temperature controller and is visualized on the front panel. There is a second thermometer with platinum resistance, or a thermocouple, to register independently the temperature–time profiles of the chamber and of the samples.

The freezing chamber consists of an open glass recipient. A fan engine, a nozzle for the dispersion of the liquid nitrogen, a thermometer with platinum resistance and a warmer are mounted on the base of the chamber. The upper part of the chamber is closed by a lid onto which 15 sample containers are hung. In one of these, it is possible to insert a probe to check the temperature of the sample. The lid is connected to a steel tube which has its lower extremity near the fan in order to assure both a uniform circulation of the nitrogen gas and a uniform temperature. The samples are mounted on the appropriate supports, which can be individually removed. Each position is sealed by a nylon plug and fixed with a safety device.

The pressure pump must be connected and firmly fixed to the nitrogen container with the appropriate hooks. It is necessary to close the valve and press the button which activates the warming in order to reach the right pressure. It is also necessary to check if the tank contains enough liquid nitrogen to complete the freezing cycle and that the pressure does not exceed the values of 0.25–0.50 bar. When the freezing is finished, it is essential to open the safety valve in order to reset the pressure. It is very dangerous to leave the pump in pressure.

As regards maintenance, it is done carefully by cleaning the inside of the freezing chamber in order to avoid damage to the electric valve on the base. It is important to verify that there is no material inside the chamber which could interfere with the functioning of the electric valve.

Rapid thawing

There are four thawing solutions, each containing decreasing cryoprotectant molarity. The thawing procedure is the same for all the solutions described above.

Methodology

Start taking out the straw from the liquid nitrogen and keep it:
1. 30 seconds in air (RT).
2. 40 seconds in water-bath at 30 °C.
3. Cut the straw at one end with sterile scissors and fix the insulin type syringe at this end.
4. Cut the other end and pour the liquid into thawing solution 1 and visualize the oocytes with the microscope.
5. Move the samples from one solution to another following the scheme.

Volume, temperature and time of exposure during rapid thawing

SOLUTION	VOLUME	INCUBATION TIME	TEMPERATURE
Sol. 1: 1.0 M PROH + 0.3 M sucrose + 30% DSS	0.5 ml	5 min	RT
Sol. 2: 0.5 M PROH + 0.3 M sucrose + 30% DSS	0.5 ml	5 min	RT
Sol. 3: 0.3 M sucrose + 30% DSS	0.5 ml	10 min	RT
Sol. 4: PBS + 30% DSS	0.5 ml	10 min	RT
Sol. 4: PBS + 30% DSS	0.5 ml	10 min	37 °C

RT = room temperature.

At the end of procedure, put the samples in 4 wells Nunclon with culture medium and oil. Leave the oocytes in culture until insemination. Figure 5.7 shows the 4 wells Nunclon prepared for thawing.

Prepare a water-bath at 30 °C and a small container filled with liquid nitrogen. Trace the samples, remove them from the dewar and immerse them in the small container of liquid nitrogen. Provide sterile scissors, sterile gauze, a watch and a report with incubation times indicated, Pasteur pipette and a syringe with an adaptor.

Choose the straw to be thawed and remove it from the nitrogen after checking the time. Keep the straw in air for 30 seconds and then keep it immersed for 40 seconds in the water-bath at 30 °C. Remove it from the water and dry it with sterile gauze. Cut an extremity and connect the syringe filled with air. Cut the other extremity and empty the contents into the well containing the first thawing solution. This operation must be done using the

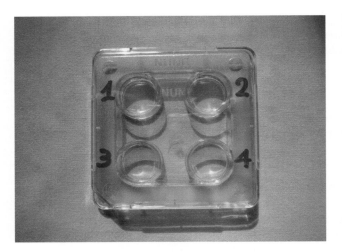

Figure 5.7 4 wells Nunclon prepared for thawing.

	Surname, Name Oocyte number			
5 minutes Solution 1				
5 minutes Solution 2				
10 minutes Solution 3				
10 minutes (RT) Solution 4				
10 minutes 37 °C Solution 4				
Culture				

Figure 5.8 Time table used to monitor times of incubation in the thawing solutions.

microscope so that the oocytes can be visualized immediately. As soon as they are detected, write the time on the report. This is the starting time of the procedure. The other times are calculated from this moment and the end is Time 0 which is the start of culture. When the thawing is concluded, the surviving oocytes are put in a Petri dish with culture medium and oil, to wait for the insemination. It is possible to thaw more than one straw at one time, depending on operator experience.

Oocyte degeneration can take place in any one of these passages. It can happen when the oocytes leak from the straw, during the thawing steps, at Time 0 and during the culture before insemination. Naturally, if degeneration is early, it is possible to immediately begin thawing other oocytes; on the contrary, if it is late (it is discovered at the moment of the ICSI), it is necessary to start the thawing operation again. The degeneration is principally identified by observing the color and consistency of the cytoplasm, which appears dark, gray and is not tridimensional. The absence of the perivitelline space, due to oolemma rupture, can be observed. Ruptures of the zona pellucida can rarely be observed.

Figure 5.8 shows the time table used to monitor the incubation times into the thawing solutions.

| Surname, Name | | | | | | | | Date and Place of birth | | | | | |

OOCYTES				PN	EMBRYOS DAY 2			EMBRYOS DAY 3			FATE		
					Time			Check time					
N° OO	Post-thawing quality	Nuclear maturity	ICSI time	Time post-ICSI	N° of blastomeres % of fragments	Grade	Note	N° of blastomeres % fragments	Grade	Note	Trans	Freezing	Discarded
Signature			Signature	Signature	Signature			Signature				Signature	

NOTES _____

Date of freezing ____/____/____ N° thawing cycle ____ N° of frozen oocytes left ____ End of thawing (time) ___:___

Culture medium, Lot N°, date of expiry_____

Embryo transfer (Embryologist/Gynecologist) _____

Transfer time ____:____

Figure 5.9 Laboratory report used to register the data of a thawing cycle from the oocytes thawing to the embryo transfer.

Times required for the entire procedure

Time required for freezing solutions' preparation: 40 minutes.

Time required for the preparation of a freezing cycle (choose the modality of division of the samples in the straws, preparation of the 4 wells Nunclon, time for the solutions to achieve room temperature, preparation of the device used for identification [jonc], preparation of storage devices [goblet, metal stick], choose the storage position [dewar and canister number], notation of the data on paper and in the computer registers, preparation and loading of the pressure pump, time necessary to reach the starting temperature of the instrument): 40 minutes.

The time required for incubation and loading of the samples varies from 20 minutes to 35 minutes. This time can change with a variation in the number of oocytes that must be frozen in that cycle. Freezing an excessive number of oocytes per cycle whilst not exceeding these times is recommended.

Total duration of the freezing program: 1 hour 50 minutes; storage: 5 minutes.

Total time: 215 minutes (230 minutes).

Time required for thawing solution preparation: 40 minutes.

The time required for the preparation of the 4 wells Nunclon, the time for the solutions to achieve room temperature, updating the data in the register and on the database and to trace the samples requires about 30 minutes. The thawing procedure of a straw (which contains from one to three oocytes) requires 45 minutes. The breaks included in the procedure permit the simultaneous thawing of more than one straw depending on the operator's experience. Figure 5.9 shows the report used to register the data of the thawing cycle and check the behavior of the thawed oocytes from thawing until the moment of embryo transfer.

Vitrification

Principles

The concept of vitrification goes back to 1937. Luney affirmed that the formation of ice crystals is incompatible with life and that the freezing of small living systems is possible only if performed at high speed, to allow the creation of a state similar to glass. During vitrification, the composition of the cellular solutions is unchanged and water does not form ice crystals.

In nature, some arctic animals adopt vitrification as a natural form of cryopreservation. It consists of a change of phase (liquid–solid) of a solution in which water acquires a phase similar to glass (amorphous) and not a crystalline phase. The viscosity of the solution, at low temperatures, becomes so high that it immobilizes the sample, which will no longer be liquid but will take on the characteristics of a solid. The conditions necessary for realizing vitrification are an elevated concentration of the cryoprotectants and an elevated rate of cooling (15 000–30 000 °C/min). The speed at which cold temperature is conducted can be increased by the reduction in the volume of the liquid in which the sample is contained. The reduction in the volume, with a consequent increase of the rate of cooling, also allows the reduction in the concentration of the cryoprotectants and, therefore, the reduction in their potential toxicity.

$$\text{Probability of vitrification} = \frac{\text{cooling rate} \times \text{viscosity}}{\text{volume}}.$$

The rate of cooling is the principal parameter but it is not the only important factor. The chemical composition of the solutions, the time of exposure and the physical characteristics of the storage device are also fundamental.

Evolution of the vitrification technique

The first attempts at vitrification of human oocytes produced very variable (from 4% to 75%) data in terms of survival (Trounson, 1986; Al-Hasani et al., 1987; Pensis et al., 1989). Today vitrification is still not a completely standardized technique. The variables are the type and concentration of the cryoprotectants, temperature and time of exposure, and storage devices. In past years, different types of damage have been observed in the various components of the oocyte after vitrification, while, probably thanks to the recent modifications brought to the technique, recent studies have shown that this technique can be less traumatic than slow freezing.

Recent studies have faced the phenomenon of the increase in intracellular calcium in the oocytes exposed to cryoprotectants. This problem, even if in practice it has been overcome with the use of intracytoplasmic sperm injection (ICSI), has the effect of creating oocytes which have already begun their activation process before being fertilized, with probable consequences on successive development.

In a study carried out on mouse oocytes (Larman *et al.*, 2006), it was observed that the most commonly used cryoprotectants for vitrification, dimethyl sulfoxide (DMSO) and ethylene glycol, cause a notable increase in the concentration of intracellular calcium, causing the phenomenon of zona hardening. The removal of calcium from vitrification solutions does not influence the effect caused by DMSO, while it notably influences the effect caused by ethylene glycol, and it is therefore recommended (Larman *et al.*, 2006; Gardner *et al.*, 2007).

In the literature, samples have been exposed to cryoprotectants at different temperatures varying from room temperature (RT) to 37 °C in different combinations. For example: vitrification/warming RT/RT (Kuwayama *et al.*, 2005; Liebermann *et al.*, 2006), vitrification/warming RT/37 °C (Hong *et al.*, 1999; Kuwayama *et al.*, 2005; Selman *et al.*, 2006), and vitrification/warming 37 °C/37 °C (Kuleshova *et al.*, 1999; Yoon *et al.*, 2003; Gardner *et al.*, 2007; Larman *et al.*, 2007b). Numerous studies do not report, or just partially report, the temperatures used during the procedures.

The storage devices are numerous and they vary from high safety system to open systems with direct contact of the sample with the liquid nitrogen. For example:

Closed: in straw dilution (ISD), high safety open pulled straw (OPS), Cryotip, High Security Vitrification Kit (HSV).

Open: electron microscopic grid, copper grid, OPS, Flexipet denuding pipettes (FDP), hemistraw system, cryoloop, Cryotop, Cryoleaf.

The use of slush-liquid nitrogen (SN2) is also described. It is liquid nitrogen which, refrigerated in a vacuum (6500 Pa for 15 minutes), reaches the temperature of -205 °C to -210 °C. In this way, nitrogen in the form of a slush is obtained; its advantage is the reduced formation of beads of air around the device when it is dipped into the liquid nitrogen, making the process of cooling faster and allowing a reduction in the concentration of the cryoprotectants used (Risco *et al.*, 2007; Yoon *et al.*, 2007). In the literature, this method has a few clinical applications (Yoon *et al.*, 2007). It seems to be useful in the cryopreservation of micro-manipulated embryos (assisted hatching, pre-implantation genetic diagnosis, and transfer of the nucleus) (Lee *et al.*, 2007).

Vitrification/warming

Working conditions

The preparation of all solutions has to be done under laminar flow, and during the procedures reduced artificial light conditions are also advised.

Materials

REAGENTS FOR SOLUTIONS	
HAM'S F10	GIBCO
Dextran serum supplement (DSS)	Irvine Scientific, Santa Ana, California, USA
ETHYLENE GLYCOL (EG)	Sigma–Aldrich Steinheim, Germany
DIMETHYL SULFOXIDE (DMSO)	Sigma–Aldrich Steinheim, Germany
SUCROSE (SUC), m.wt. 342.3	Sigma–Aldrich Steinheim, Germany

TOOLS FOR VITRIFICATION

CRYOTIP *	Irvine Scientific, Santa Ana, California, USA
High Security Vitrification Kit (HSV) *	Cryo Bio System, IMV Technologies, France
CRYOTOP *	Kitazato BioPharma Co., Japan
Label Printer (for HSV)	LABPAL, Brady, Malaysia
SYMS-TYPE Thermal Sealer (for HSV)	Cryo Bio System, IMV Technologies, France
Impulse Bag Sealer SK-210 (for Cryotip)	Falc Instruments, Italy
DENUDING CAPILLARY 140 µl	COOK, Australia
GOBLET diameter 12 mm	Cryo Bio System, IMV Technologies, France
GOBLET diameter 65 mm	Cryo Bio System, IMV Technologies, France
METAL STICK	Cryo Bio System, IMV Technologies, France
TIMER	

* Three types of devices are indicated.

DISPOSABLE MATERIALS

STERILE TIPS FOR GILSON PIPETTE	
STERILE TIPS 1 ml	Falcon, Becton Dickinson, NJ, USA
STERILE TIPS 10 ml	Falcon, Becton Dickinson, NJ, USA
PETRI DISH 65 mm	Falcon, Becton Dickinson, NJ, USA
DENUDING CAPILLARY 140	COOK, Australia

Vitrification solutions for human oocyte

There are three vitrification solutions. The first one is a wash solution (WS), the second is a dehydration solution (equilibration solution = ES), the third one is a dehydration and loading solution (vitrification solution = VS).

Prepare the solutions in Falcon Tube 13 ml.

SOLUTION	COMPOSITION/PREPARATION
WASH SOLUTION (WS)	**HAM'S F10 + 20% DSS** 8 ml Ham's F10 + 2 ml DSS
EQUILIBRATION SOLUTION (ES)	**1.05 M DMSO + 1.35 M EG + 20% DSS** (7.5% DMSO + 7.5% EG + 20% DSS) 6.5 ml Ham's F10 + 0.75 ml DMSO + 0.75 ml EG + 2 ml DSS
VITRIFICATION SOLUTION (VS)	**2.1 M DMSO + 2.7 M EG + 0.5 M SUC + 20% DSS** (15% DMSO + 15% EG + 0.5 M SUC + 20% DSS) 1.7115 g SUC + 4 ml Ham's F10 to solubilize and then add 1.5 ml DMSO + 1.5 ml EG; make up to a volume of 8ml with Ham's F10. Add 2 ml DSS

Filter the final solutions in a new Falcon Tube 13 ml and divide them in to aliquots of 1 ml in cryovials (NUNC). Store at $+4\,^{\circ}$C.

Warming solutions for human oocytes

There are three warming solutions, which contain decreasing concentrations of sucrose. Prepare the solutions in Falcon Tube 13 ml.

SOLUTION	COMPOSITION/PREPARATION
THAWING SOLUTION (TS)	**1.0 M sucrose + 20% DSS** 3.423 g SUC + 5 ml Ham's F10 to solubilize; make up to a volume of 8ml with Ham's F10. Add 2 ml DSS
DILUENT SOLUTION (DS)	**0.5 M sucrose + 20% DSS** 1.7115 g SUC + 5 ml Ham's F10 to solubilize; make up to a volume of 8ml with Ham's F10. Add 2 ml DSS
WASH SOLUTION (WS)	**buffered medium + 20% DSS** 8 ml Ham's F10 + 2 ml DSS

Filter the final solutions in to a new Falcon Tube 13 ml and divide them in aliquots of 1 ml in cryovials (NUNC). Store at $+4\,^{\circ}$C. Vitrification and warming solutions have to be filtered starting from the less to higher concentrated one. The solutions can be stored and utilized for 60 days from the day of preparation if they are stored correctly. The day of preparation is utilized as the LOT Number.

TOOLS FOR WARMING	
STERILE SCISSORS	
TIMER	
AUTOMATIC INSULATION STRIPPER (KNIPEX, Germany)	

DISPOSABLE MATERIALS FOR WARMING	
STERILE TIPS	
DENUDING CAPILLARY	COOK, Australia
PETRI DISH 65 mm	FALCON, Becton Dickinson, NJ, USA

Devices for vitrification

Three types of devices will be described in detail. The mode of utilization during the phases of vitrification and warming will also be reported.

Figure 6.1 shows the High Security Vitrification Kit (HSV). It is formed by a gutter-like hemistraw and by a high security straw. An introducer is provided to help during the insertion and extraction of the hemistraw.

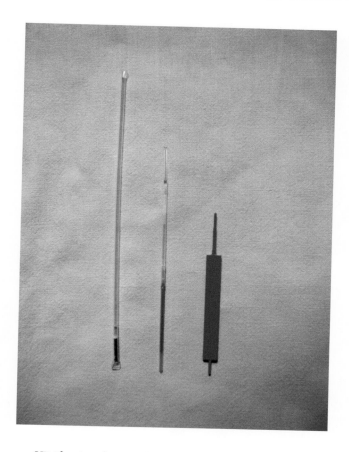

Figure 6.1 High Security Vitrification Kit (HSV) (Cryo Bio System, IMV Technologies, France).

Vitrification: the sample is loaded in a volume lower than 0.2 µl on the terminal part of the hemistraw. After the sample loading, the hemistraw is immediately inserted into the high security straw using an introducer. The straw is immediately sealed using an appropriate sealer (SYMS-type thermal sealer, Cryo Bio System). The sample must be vitrified by plunging the device into liquid nitrogen in less than one minute from the moment of exposure to the VS solution. The device must maintain a circular movement for at least one minute in the liquid nitrogen before storage. The circular movement prevents the formation of air bubbles around the device at the moment of immersion that could slow down the rate of cooling.

Warming: keeping the device in the liquid nitrogen, the high security straw is cut with sterile scissors or an automatic insulation stripper. The hemistraw is taken out by the help of the introducer and it is immediately immersed into the thawing solution (TS) at 37 °C. Usually the sample comes out alone from the gutter, but sometimes the denuding pipette is used to help it out. It is very easy to localize the sample with a microscope.

Figure 6.2 shows the Cryotip device (Irvine Scientific, Santa Ana, California). It consists of a plastic straw with a thin part connected to a thicker and wider part and provided with a sliding protective metallic sleeve.

Vitrification: the sample is loaded on the thick side of the device in about 1 microliter of solution without air bubbles, as a result of aspiration using a syringe connected to the

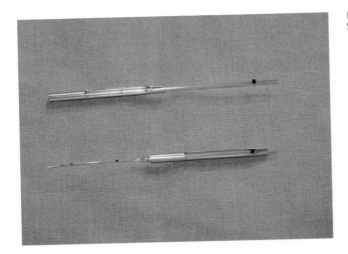

Figure 6.2 Cryotip (Irvine Scientific, Santa Ana, California).

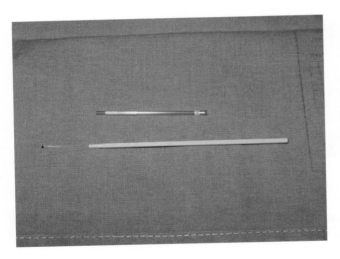

Figure 6.3 Cryotop (Kitazato BioPharma Co., Japan).

device. The Cryotip is sealed at both ends and the sleeve is pulled towards the thin side. The device is plunged into liquid nitrogen. The time required to load the sample, prepare the sleeve and immerse the device in liquid nitrogen does not exceed one minute.

Warming: the Cryotip is removed from the liquid nitrogen and immediately immersed in a water-bath at 37 °C, dried with sterile gauze, and cut using sterile scissors. The contents are poured into the TS at 37 °C. Oocytes are easily localized with a microscope.

Figure 6.3 illustrates the Cryotop device (Kitazato BioPharma Co., Japan), which consists of a polypropylene strip attached to a plastic part and fitted with a cap.

Vitrification: each sample is loaded in very small volumes (<0.1 μl "minimal volume") on the extreme side of the tip just before the black mark. The Cryotop is plunged in to "filtered" liquid nitrogen, keeping it moving for a few seconds. While the Cryotop remains immersed, the cap is attached with the aid of forceps.

Warming: the cap is removed while the device is immersed in the liquid nitrogen. The terminal part of the Cryotop is immediately immersed into the TS at 37 °C. Usually the samples peel off from the strip and they are easily localized with a microscope.

Mode of utilization of the devices during vitrification phase
Mode of utilization of HSV during vitrification phase

The following sequence of images, Figures 6.4–6.11, shows the correct use of the HSV during vitrification. The identification of the HSV is made by means of labels which have previously been prepared using a specific printer (LABPAL, Brady, Malaysia).

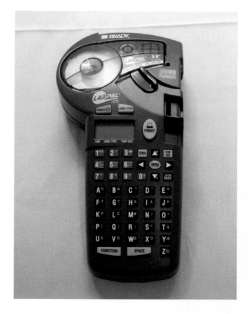

Figure 6.4 Label printer.

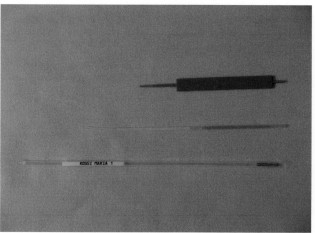

Figure 6.5 HSV identification.

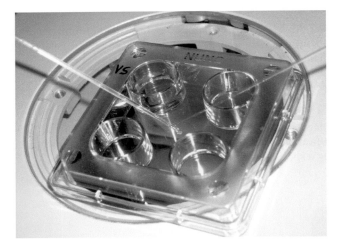

Figure 6.6 HSV sample loading.

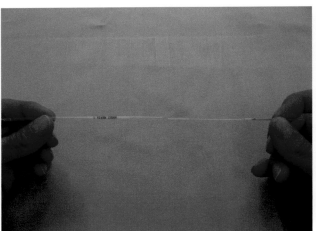

Figure 6.7 Hemistraw insertion into the security straw.

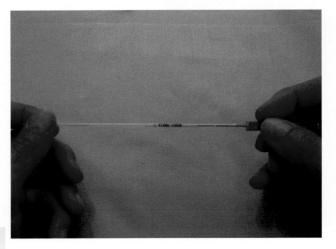

Figure 6.8 Use of the introducer for the complete introduction of the hemistraw.

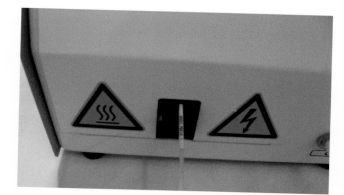

Figure 6.9 Thermal sealer.

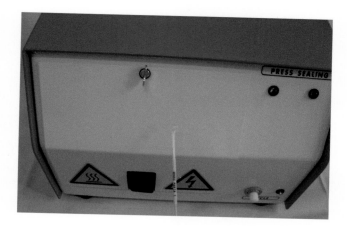

Figure 6.10 The sealed HSV.

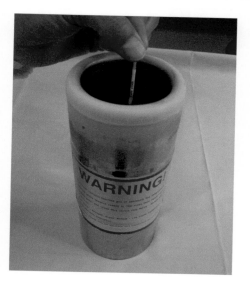

Figure 6.11 Plunging the straw into liquid nitrogen. Maintain a circular movement for about one minute.

Mode of utilization of Cryotip during vitrification phase

The following sequence of images, Figures 6.12–6.16, shows the correct use of the Cryotip during vitrification.

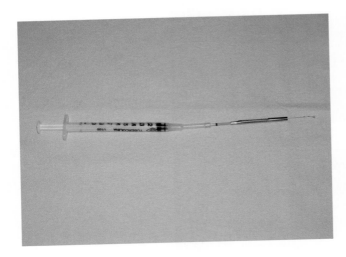

Figure 6.12 Cryotip connected to the insulin type syringe by a silicone tube.

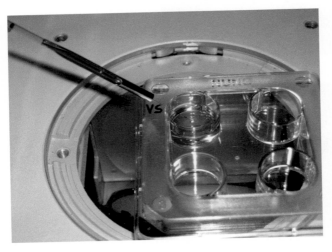

Figure 6.13 Cryotip during sample loading.

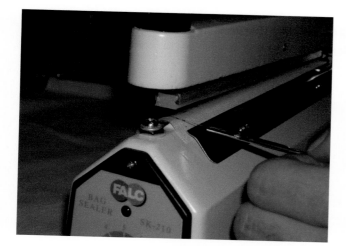

Figure 6.14 Sealing of the thin side of the straw.

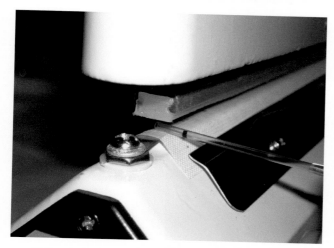

Figure 6.15 Sealing of the thick side of the straw.

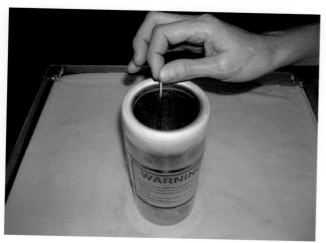

Figure 6.16 Plunging the straw into liquid nitrogen. Maintain a circular movement for about one minute.

Mode of utilization of Cryotop during vitrification phase

The following sequence of images, Figures 6.17–6.20, shows the correct use of the Cryotop during vitrification.

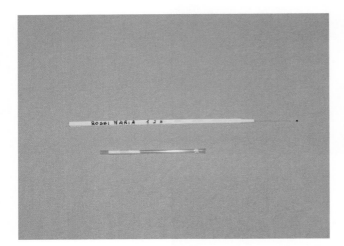

Figure 6.17 Cryotop identification.

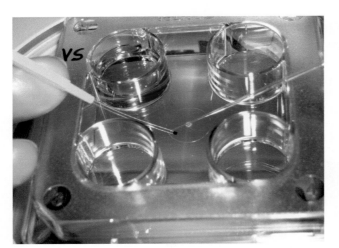

Figure 6.18 Cryotop loading.

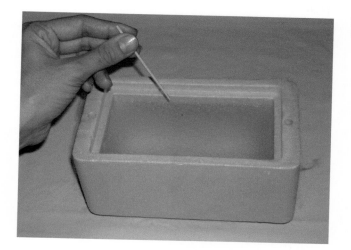

Figure 6.19 Cryotop plunging into liquid nitrogen.

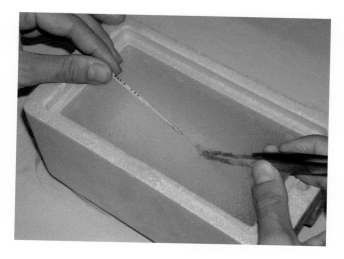

Figure 6.20 Cryotop cap affixing.

Method of storing

The method of storing is the same for all the cryopreservation techniques. An identified metal stick is prepared. Two goblets (12 mm diameter) are utilized. One of them is cut to make a cap for the other. The goblet containing the samples is attached to the metal stick and stored in the dewar. The metal stick and the goblet are identified. Figures 6.21 and 6.22 show the method of storage for the different cryopreservation techniques (slow freezing and vitrification). Figure 6.21 shows a metal stick and two goblets. One of them is used to create a cap. The goblet with the cap held by the metal stick is also shown. Figure 6.22 shows identified goblets with the accompanying metal stick inside the dewar of storage.

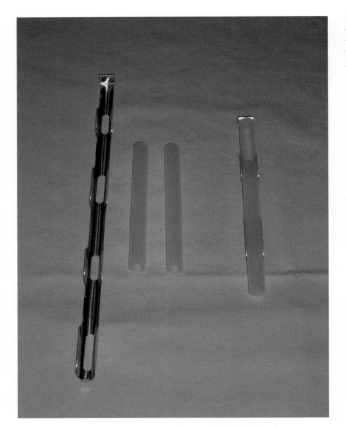

Figure 6.21 One metal stick and two goblets. One of them is used to create a cap. The goblet with the cap held by the metal stick is also shown.

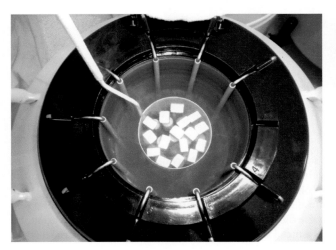

Figure 6.22 Identified goblets with the metal stick inside the dewar of storage.

Mode of utilization of the devices during warming phase

Mode of utilization of the HSV during warming phase

The following sequence of images, Figures 6.23–6.26, shows the correct use of the HSV during the warming procedure.

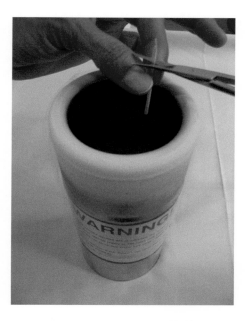

Figure 6.23 Cut off the security straw. The HSV is still immersed in the liquid nitrogen.

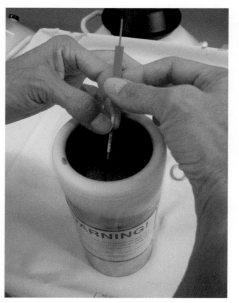

Figure 6.24 Starting of the hemistraw extraction with the help of the introducer.

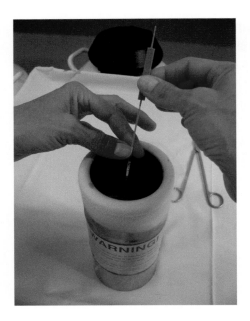

Figure 6.25 Hemistraw extraction with the help of introducer.

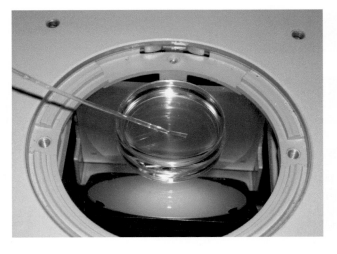

Figure 6.26 HSV sample recovery into thawing solution at 37 °C.

Mode of utilization of the Cryotip during warming phase

The following sequence of images, Figures 6.27–6.29, shows the correct use of the Cryotip during warming.

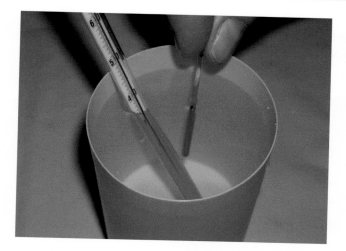

Figure 6.27 Cryotip immersion in 37 °C water-bath immediately after removal from liquid nitrogen.

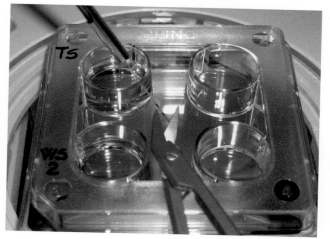

Figure 6.28 Cut of the thin side of the straw.

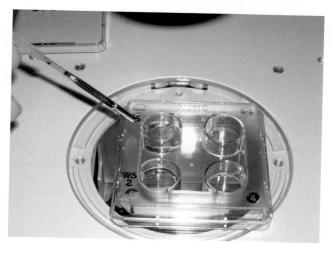

Figure 6.29 Samples recovery in thawing solution at 37 °C.

Mode of utilization of the Cryotop during warming phase

The following sequence of images, Figures 6.30 and 6.31, shows the correct use of the Cryotop during warming.

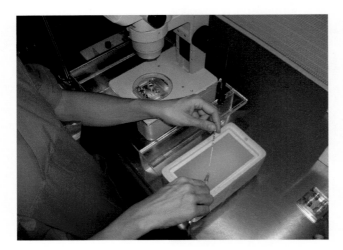

Figure 6.30 Cryotop cup extraction into the liquid nitrogen.

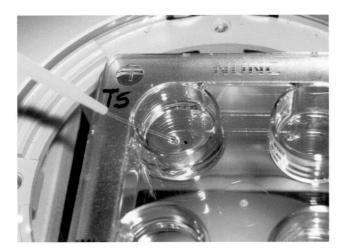

Figure 6.31 Cryotop sample recovery into thawing solution at 37 °C.

Vitrification

The procedure described (Kuwayama, 2007) was slightly modified in our laboratory. Keep the solutions out of the refrigerator and leave them at RT. Utilize a Petri dish (65 mm) and one 4 wells Nunclon for each device that you have arranged.

Make a big (60 μl) and a small (20 μl) drop of WS (WS1, WS2). Make three drops (20 μl) of ES (ES1, ES2, ES3). Put 0.5 ml of VS into one well. Figure 6.32 shows the Petri dish set for vitrification and the sequence of utilization. The drop volume is 20 μl.

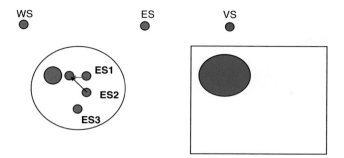

Figure 6.32 Preparation of Petri dish and sequence of use for vitrification. The drop volume is 20 µl.

SOLUTION	INCUBATION TIME	TEMPERATURE
WS1	Wash sample from oil	RT
WS2	10 sec	RT
ES1	3 min	RT
ES2	3 min	RT
ES3	Max 9 min	RT
VS	4 washes (5 sec each)	RT

RT = room temperature.

Vitrification procedure

Take the sample using a 140 µl denuding pipette and put it in the big drop of WS. Take the sample and put it into the small drop of WS, being careful not to drag oil, which could be a problem during the successive operations. Watch the oocyte, noting its morphology and, above all, the width of its perivitelline space.

Join the ES1 drop to the WS using a sterile tip. Start the timer (3 minutes). Join the ES2 drop to the WS using a sterile tip. Start the timer (3 minutes). The arrows in Figure 6.32 indicate the way to join the drops. Transfer the sample ES3 using a 140 µl denuding pipette. Start the timer and watch the oocyte. Stop the incubation when the perivitelline space returns to its original dimensions, with a maximum incubation time of 9 minutes.

Take the sample and transfer it to a Petri dish containing VS. Wash it rapidly by moving it inside the dish at least four times. Incubation in VS must be very quick because the sample has to be vitrified within one minute.

Take the oocyte and load it in to the chosen device in as small a volume as possible. Utilize the base of the 4 wells Nunclon to load the sample on the device (for HSV and Cryotop). Proceed immediately with vitrification. If an open device is used, immerse it immediately in liquid nitrogen; if a closed device is used, seal it rapidly and then plunge it into liquid nitrogen. Figures 6.33–6.37 show the sequence of steps during the incubation of samples in vitrification solutions.

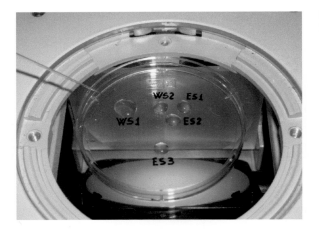

Figure 6.33 Petri dish set for vitrification.

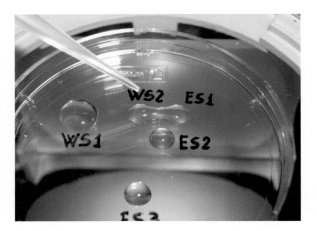

Figure 6.34 ES1 joined to WS2.

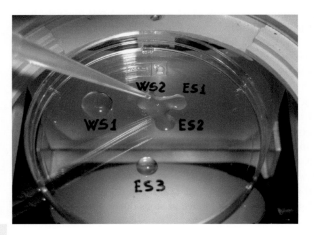

Figure 6.35 ES2 joined to WS2.

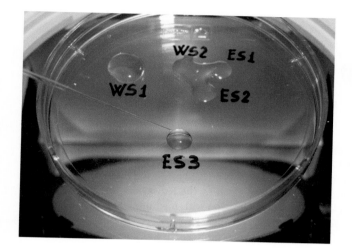

Figure 6.36 Incubation in ES3.

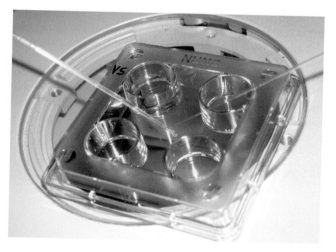

Figure 6.37 Sample loading device.

Minimum volume

This concept means that the sample has to be loaded on the device with as small a volume as possible (Kuwayama, 2007). This can be done by loading the sample in a small volume and leaving it at the tip of the denuding pipette. Then, the excess volume has to be taken out, aspirating it with the denuding pipette until the sample is covered only by a thin layer of liquid. This concept is very important because the smaller the volume, the quicker and more efficacious will be the vitrification process.

Warming procedure

The procedure described by Kuwayama (2007) was slightly modified in our laboratory. Keep the solution out of the refrigerator. Put TS at 37 °C while diluent solution (DS) and WS are at RT. Utilize two 4 wells Nunclon as follows (they are enough for the warming of two devices).

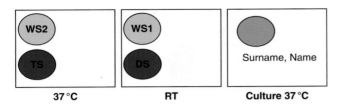

Put an aliquot of 0.8 ml of TS and 0.5 ml of WS (WS2) into separate wells of the 4 wells Nunclon and keep them at 37 °C.

Put an aliquot of 0.5 ml of DS and 0.5 ml of WS (WS1) into the other 4 well and keep them at RT. These temperatures are those indicated by the Kuwayama method.

Furthermore, prepare an identified 4 well Nunclon with medium and oil for the culture. Put it in the incubator (one for each patient).

Figure 6.38 shows the preparation of the 4 wells Nunclon and the sequence of utilization of warming solutions.

Open the device and take it out from the liquid nitrogen as previously indicated in the details for each device. Recover the sample by plunging the device in TS at 37 °C. Localize the sample, focusing the microscope, and start the timer. From this moment utilize a 140 μl denuding pipette to move the sample from one solution to the other.

Leave in TS for 1 minute. Keep the sample in a little amount of TS with a capillary and leave it in DS at RT for 3 minutes. Keep the sample in a little amount of DS and leave it in WS1 at RT for 5 minutes. Keep the sample in a little amount of WS1 and leave it in WS2 at RT for 1 minute. Keep the sample and put the survived samples in culture until ICSI.

SOLUTION	INCUBATION TIME	TEMPERATURE
TS	1 min	37 °C
DS	3 min	RT
WS1	5 min	RT
WS2	1 min	RT
CULTURE	Until ICSI	37 °C

RT = room temperature.

The passage from one solution to another is carried out by keeping the oocytes in a small quantity of the solution in which they are found and releasing them into the next solution. In this way, the passage between the different molarities becomes less shocking.

The temperature of exposition during the procedures

The temperature of exposition during the vitrification and warming procedures represents a debated and non-standardized topic. In the literature, the conditions and combinations of RT and 37 °C are reported.

In addition to this, the term RT is not codified. In fact, according to some authors, it corresponds to 22–23 °C and for other authors to 25–27 °C. These differences are very important both for cryoprotectant exposition and for meiotic spindle behavior, which is very sensitive to temperature variations. Our center has carried out some studies regarding this topic. We compared meiotic spindle behavior in slow freezing/thawing at RT (22–23 °C) with the behavior during vitrification/warming at different temperature combinations: RT/RT (22–23 °C); RT (22–23 °C)/37 °C; 37 °C/37 °C. The results demonstrated that vitrification is associated with a faster recovery of the meiotic spindle after warming compared to slow freezing and that the fastest recovery in vitrification is associated with 37 °C/37 °C; in the latter conditions, the results show that a considerable proportion of the oocytes maintain the meiotic spindle without depolymerization. The oocytes which are not exposed to non-physiological temperatures do not, or only slightly, undergo spindle depolymerization (Ciotti *et al.*, 2009). Other authors confirm these observations (Gardner *et al.*, 2007; Larman *et al.*, 2007b). Kuwayama reports optimal clinical results, mainly using RT (25–27 °C) and using a temperature of 37 °C (TS) only during the first and the last step of warming. Our center is carrying out an internal comparative study to establish the best temperature in the different phases. We are using the conditions indicated by Kuwayama and the three conditions described in our study (Ciotti *et al.*, 2009).

Liquid nitrogen filtration

The problem of liquid nitrogen filtration arises in the case of vitrification using "open" devices, because the biological samples are in direct contact with the liquid nitrogen. In these cases, a certain quantity of nitrogen (about 500 ml for each patient) is filtered; this nitrogen will be used for the immersion of the device at the moment of vitrification.

In this way, we obtain filtration but not sterilization. The filters used are 0.2 micrometers; therefore, viruses and mycoplasma can pass through the filter. Furthermore, it is not exactly known if the filter can weather the extreme temperature of –196 °C. The filters used are made of Teflon because this seems to be the most resistant material at low temperatures. Omnipore filters (Millipore, Ireland) are put into envelopes and sterilized at 120 °C for 20 minutes. They are applied to a glass filtration system (Millipore). This is formed by a glass container, a connecting part with a porous surface on which the sterile filter is positioned, and an upper part in which the liquid nitrogen is poured. A metal pincer is utilized to keep the different parts together. The nitrogen is poured into the upper container. The system is connected to an aspiration pump that creates a negative pressure which aspirates the nitrogen through the filter placing it into the lower flask. The glass system is kept in a box partially filled with liquid nitrogen during utilization. Figures 6.39–6.41 show the procedure for liquid nitrogen filtration.

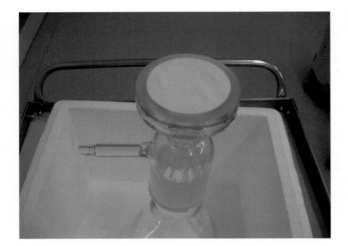

Figure 6.39 Sterile Omnipore filter positioned on filter unit.

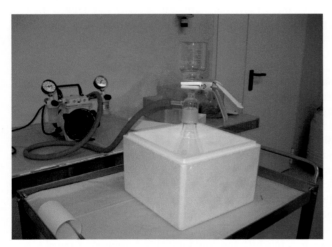

Figure 6.40 Glass filter unit connected to the pressure pump.

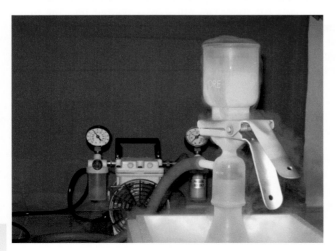

Figure 6.41 Filter unit filled with liquid nitrogen while the pump is working.

During the procedure the operator must wear protective clothing for handling liquid nitrogen (gloves, mask) and it is necessary to maintain good ventilation because of the notable dispersion of liquid nitrogen. In fact, it is necessary to use a quantity of nitrogen three times larger than the volume required for the final result.

Time needed for the entire procedure (vitrification and warming)

The preparation of the vitrification solutions requires about 40 minutes.

The preparation of the material, the decision about sample subdivision into the devices, the identification of the devices, the decision on the storage position and the data registration require approximately 30 minutes. The procedure of nitrogen filtration requires approximately one hour. One or two oocytes are placed in each device. The time necessary to complete the vitrification of a device varies from 13 minutes to 17 minutes. This time must be multiplied by the number of devices to be vitrified.

The preparation of the warming solutions requires approximately 40 minutes.

The preparation of the material, the recovery of the samples, the updating of the data in the register and on the database requires approximately 20 minutes.

The warming of a device requires 14 minutes. This time must be multiplied by the number of devices which require warming.

PolScope evaluation after cryopreservation procedures

By using PolScope, it is possible to evaluate the presence of the meiotic spindle during the procedures as well as at the end and at different times after the end in order to determine the time of the reappearance of the spindle. It is possible to compare the image of the spindle taken before cryopreservation with the one taken after the procedure and to establish if it has reacquired its original retardance. When the presence of the meiotic spindle has been verified, it is possible to proceed with ICSI.

Comparison between slow freezing and vitrification: pros and cons

Introduction

A study carried out by Gardner *et al.* (2007) points out the importance of evaluating membrane permeability and physiology for the success of oocyte cryopreservation, and gives indications about the most recent scientific tendencies, although these are based on animal oocytes or embryos. The experiments show that slow freezing results in a greater reduction in the oxidative metabolism and of the utilization of nutrients compared with vitrification. In addition to this, vitrification does not result in loss of lactic dehydrogenase (marker of membrane integrity). In conclusion, vitrification has a lower impact on the energetic metabolism and on membrane integrity compared with slow freezing. Proteomic analysis also gives better results for vitrification; in fact, slow freezing seems to be associated with larger alterations which happen in the cooling period before the seeding due to the long exposition to 1,2-propanediol (PROH).

Another important aspect is related to the meiotic spindle. As we know, its integrity is fundamental for the correct function of all the developing events that follow fertilization of the oocyte. It is equally known that it is very sensitive to temperature changes, according to its protein structure. The decreasing temperature influences very strictly the meiotic spindle organization, and its preservation represents one of the most important factors that determine the success of the cryopreservation.

Many studies have underlined the meiotic spindle's cryovulnerability (Pickering and Johnson, 1987; Sathananthan *et al.*, 1988; Pickering *et al.*, 1990; van Der Elst *et al.*, 1992; Boiso *et al.*, 2002) and its plasticity, that is, its capacity of reformation if it is exposed to physiological temperatures after freezing (Pickering and Johnson, 1987; Gook *et al.*, 1993; Cobo *et al.*, 2001). Furthermore, other authors have found normal karyotypes and the absence of dispersed chromosomes after the fertilization of thawed oocytes (Gook *et al.*, 1994; Cobo *et al.*, 2001). The invasive studies gave only a static and isolated image of the meiotic spindle structure and, by impeding the successive use of the oocyte, impeded an evaluation of its developmental capacity. Recently, thanks to the introduction of an instrument called a PolScope (Oldenbourg, 1996; Keefe *et al.*, 2003), which uses the characteristics of polarized light, it has become possible to study in vivo the dynamic behavior of the spindle during cooling (Wang *et al.*, 2001) and during cryopreservation procedures (Rienzi *et al.*, 2004; Bianchi *et al.*, 2005). Studies carried out during dehydration and rehydration procedures for slow freezing have demonstrated that exposure to cryoprotectants stabilizes the spindle, which remains clearly visible for the entire period of incubation (Rienzi *et al.*, 2004). It was also shown that the spindle depolymerizes during the thawing phases and repolymerizes, in the majority of the oocytes, after at least three hours of culture, that is after the exposition to the physiological temperature for a few hours (Rienzi *et al.*, 2004; Bianchi *et al.*, 2005). As regards slow freezing, all the procedures are carried out at room temperature (RT) and, thus, it is normal that the meiotic spindle depolymerizes during the phase of cryoprotectant removal, which lasts about 40 minutes, and reforms after returning to 37 °C for a certain period of time. As has previously been described in the literature, many authors carry out the vitrification and warming procedures at physiological temperatures. Gardner *et al.* (2007) reported that meiotic spindle visualization is possible by observing the oocytes at the end of the warming procedure carried out at 37 °C. Another study (Larman *et al.*, 2007b) showed that carrying out the vitrification/warming of human and animal oocytes entirely at 37 °C permits the meiotic spindle to remain intact and not to have significantly altered retardance values. Instead, if the same procedure is carried out at RT (20–21 °C), the retardance is significantly diminished. Another study which sustains this thesis has been carried out in our laboratory (Ciotti *et al.*, 2009). This study had the aim of monitoring meiotic spindle behavior during and after slow freezing and vitrification, by observing the oocytes in each passage of the different procedures using the PolScope. The slow freezing/thawing was carried out at RT while the vitrification/warming was carried out at different temperatures: RT/RT, RT/37 °C, 37 °C/37 °C. The results have confirmed the meiotic spindle behavior as previously described for slow freezing and warming at RT (Rienzi *et al.*, 2004; Bianchi *et al.*, 2005). Meiotic spindle recovery was significantly faster for vitrification than for slow freezing, but in both procedures recovery took place in 100% of the oocytes observed. Temperature is a crucial element since the earliest visualization took place in the procedure which did not include exposition of the samples to non-physiological temperatures. At the end of the vitrification/warming procedure at 37 °C/37 °C, a certain percentage of oocytes showed the presence of the meiotic spindle before the end of the procedure, that is, when the oocyte, by reacquiring its original volume, became visible with the Polscope. This observation leads us to believe that the meiotic spindle does not depolymerize during the entire procedure, maintaining its original structure. This has the twofold advantage of not requiring spindle reformation and of shortening the waiting periods for oocyte insemination, by reducing the aging time in vitro. Cobo *et al.* (2008d) compared spindle repolymerization in different cryopreservation protocols: slow freezing with 0.2 M sucrose, 0.3 M sucrose, 0.3 M sucrose in sodium-depleted medium, and vitrification. The results showed that the internal structure was observed in the majority of oocytes after three hours of culture, independently of the cryopreservation technique utilized. It must be considered that the studies cited which considered meiotic spindle behavior in vitrification (Larman *et al.*, 2007b; Cobo *et al.*, 2008d; Ciotti *et al.*, 2009) were carried out using different storage systems: cryoloop, High Security Vitrification Kit (HSV), Cryotop.

The cytoskeleton can also suffer damage which can lead to problems during chromosomal segregation and during cell division, after cryopreservation. This damage seems to be more substantial during slow freezing compared to vitrification because of the long dehydration and rehydration process.

Practical advantages and disadvantages of slow freezing versus vitrification

Practical advantages and disadvantages can be found for both techniques. Slow freezing has a high initial cost for the purchase of a programmable freezer which is not necessary for vitrification. On the contrary, the devices for vitrification are more expensive than those for slow freezing.

	Slow freezing	Vitrification
Computer freezer	Yes	No
Duration of procedure	Long (even if the oocyte number is low)	Brief (if the oocyte number is low)
Operator experience	High	Very high
Type of technique	Fairly standardized	Still very variable
Cost of storage devices	Low	Very high in some cases
Cost of solutions	Elevated if bought	Elevated if bought
Average waiting time for performing ICSI	2–3 hours	1 hour
Safety of storage	Tested	To be tested

The time spent to carry out the procedures is only apparently shorter for vitrification. In fact, if we consider the time spent for nitrogen filtration and the necessity of vitrifying a large number of oocytes, the time spent for vitrification is surely longer. In addition to this, vitrification requires the constant presence of an operator until the end of the procedure. In the case of slow freezing, it is possible to freeze a large number of oocytes (even 50) in the same session without a notable increase in the time spent for incubation and loading. Moreover, after beginning the freezing program, the operator must only carry out the seeding (about 20 minutes after the start) and can carry out other activities until the program ends and the samples are ready to be stored.

In the course of the working day, slow freezing has the disadvantage of having to wait for all the oocytes destined for cryopreservation. This means that on the days in which several pickups have been scheduled, the first patients are penalized with respect to the last ones because their oocytes have longer in vitro aging. In this way, some oocytes could wait for 7–8 hours to be frozen. This is not a good practice and it could seriously compromise the results. In these cases the oocytes could be divided into two different freezing sessions with a consequent notable waste of time.

As regards vitrification instead, if an operator is expressly assigned to this activity, it is possible to vitrify the oocytes of each patient one by one following the pickup order, thus always maintaining a very short time of in vitro culture. When there are a lot of oocytes to be cryopreserved it would, however, be a good practice to spread out the vitrification procedure over the work day, both because of the previously described motive and because the work is very tiring for the operator and requires great precision and attention without distraction.

Recently, a fact in favor of vitrification has been emerging: the reduced or absent depolymerization of the meiotic spindle. In addition to the theoretical advantage of preserving the original spindle without requiring a reformation process which could have negative consequences, this has the practical advantage of reducing the waiting period between the end of the procedure and the intracytoplasmic sperm injection (ICSI). In fact, a waiting period of an hour, which represents the time necessary to allow the oocyte to reach equilibrium in the new condition, is sufficient before performing insemination. This aspect permits the further reduction of the time of in vitro aging.

Vitrification is associated with possible contamination when it is carried out in open devices, where the samples and the liquid nitrogen are in direct contact. For some, this is only a theoretical problem. However, even if the risk is very low, it still exists, and we must try to reduce it as much as possible. Because of this, the nitrogen is filtered, that is, cleaned, through filters (0.2 micrometers) smaller than the ones usually inserted at the end of liquid nitrogen supply (0.5 micrometers). Naturally, it would be desirable to find a closed device which gives results similar to the open ones but, at the moment, the results reported in the literature are in favor of open systems, in terms of survival, pregnancy and implantation. The vitrification of a sample is a process that can be obtained also at relatively high temperatures by increasing the cryoprotectants concentration, but it is important to reduce the volume of solution which contains the sample and increase the freezing rate in order to reduce the cytotoxic effect of the high concentration of cryoprotectants. This process is of course optimized when there are no barriers between the sample and the nitrogen.

Some patients may ask to transfer their oocytes from one center to another which creates the problem of sample transport. This problem is more important in the case of vitrified samples than frozen samples. As regards vitrification, the samples are more fragile, more sensitive to temperature changes and thus more susceptible to damage because of the minimal volume. The transport must be carried out very cautiously by specialized personnel.

The results between the two techniques are still difficult to compare. Some teams support the less traumatic qualities of slow freezing and others have completely embraced vitrification as a panacea for cryopreservation in the bounds of PMA. Our center is carrying out a parallel study to compare the two different procedures if performed by the same operators and in the same environment. However, we believe that the results depend on the characteristics of the center, operator experience and the number of operators available. Some centers could have better results by using one technique instead of the other, or some groups of patients or oocytes having particular characteristics may have better responses to one of the two techniques. As regards vitrification, discussion about which devices to use and the exposition temperature is still open. However, some modifications could also be introduced in slow freezing as, for example, optimizing the thawing phase, which has not been modified in years.

8

Safety of storage

Liquid nitrogen supply and cryocontainer fill-up

Modalities and rules for correctly supplying liquid nitrogen

Three types of cryocontainers are necessary:

1. Dewars containing biological samples.
2. Dewars of liquid nitrogen. They are attached to the pressure pump to provide nitrogen during functioning of the programmable freezer.
3. In pressure dewars. These are used to fill the above cryocontainers by attaching the specific liquid supply.

To correctly maintain the liquid biological samples in liquid nitrogen, it is necessary to insure that the cryocontainers are regularly filled up with liquid nitrogen so that the samples are always immersed. Even if the cryocontainers are closed, they disperse about 300 ml of liquid nitrogen in a week. It is, therefore, very important to maintain the liquid nitrogen levels even during the inactive periods, by organizing shifts of the staff. Our laboratory is supplied weekly with liquid nitrogen by a specific external service. The day before the delivery, the operators put the containers (under pressure and normal) in an agreed place. The following morning the service picks up the empty containers and returns them filled about two hours later.

It is very important to remember that the cryocontainers containing the biological samples always stay in the storage room. The containers provided by the external service are only nitrogen containers. The containers in pressure are obviously equipped with a security valve through which they eliminate the nitrogen gas. It is therefore necessary to carry out the operation of filling up within a few hours in order to avoid emptying of the cryocontainers in pressure. The operator must wear protective clothing (closed shoes, glasses, gloves) and must activate the security systems which assure the airing of the room in case of excessive reduction of oxygen concentration in the room. He/she must connect the specific filling supply (metal tube equipped with terminal diffuser with 0.5 micrometer pores connected to the container in pressure) to the liquid fill decant valve, open the valve and begin the fill-up of the cryocontainers.

The time required for this operation depends on the number of cryocontainers to be filled. Our laboratory presently has 20 cryocontainers. Two 60 liter containers in pressure are necessary to fill them. The complete operation requires approximately one hour.

Staff safety

Nitrogen is the most concentrated gas in the atmosphere (78%). It is an inert, colorless, odorless gas which can be liquified at $-196\,°C$. If liquid nitrogen comes into contact with the skin and the cornea in a considerable quantity, it can cause serious damage. If it is present in closed or insufficiently aired rooms, it can stratify from the bottom to the top of the room, replace the oxygen and saturate the environment very rapidly. In this case, it can cause asphyxia (air the room out immediately in order to give first aid). A percentage of oxygen lower than 18% is dangerous and lower than 10% is lethal.

The design of a cryobiological laboratory must include the possibility of locating all the instruments in a room, adjacent but separated from the PMA laboratory, which is at a controlled temperature and is provided with the possibility of aeration, an oxygen analyzer, an internal air aspirator, a ventilator (external air intake), and acoustic and visual internal and external alarms. The door of this room must be locked and only the operators should have the key to open it. The list of the operators must be available and public.

There are security norms and equipment that must be available and used by the operators handling liquid nitrogen in a cryobiological laboratory: in accordance with the European laws about security in the working environment, the company which provides the gas must provide a security card that summarizes all the characteristics of the product, whilst the employer must supply the operators with all the necessary means of avoiding physical damage.

Protection equipment

- Cryogenic gloves (resistant at low temperatures)
- Glasses
- Masks
- Fixed or portable oxygen analyzer.

Figures 8.1–8.7 show a sequence of images that show the safety devices that have to be present and functioning in a cryobiological laboratory.

Once every six months, routine maintenance of all the security systems is necessary in order to verify their correct functioning.

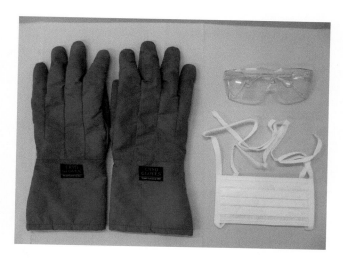

Figure 8.1 The security operator devices: cryogenic gloves, mask, and glasses.

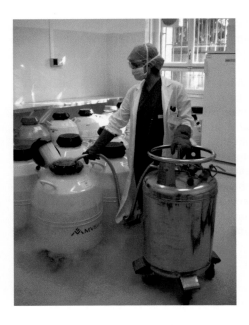

Figure 8.2 The in pressure cryocontainer attached to the specific liquid supply. The operator wears protective devices.

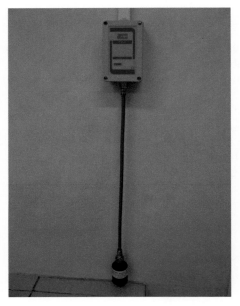

Figure 8.3 The oxygen sensor.

Directions for optimal long-term storage

To correctly maintain the samples over a period of time they must always be immersed in the liquid nitrogen, but it is also very important to pay careful attention during the execution of some processes: storage, tracing the samples at the moment of thawing, the

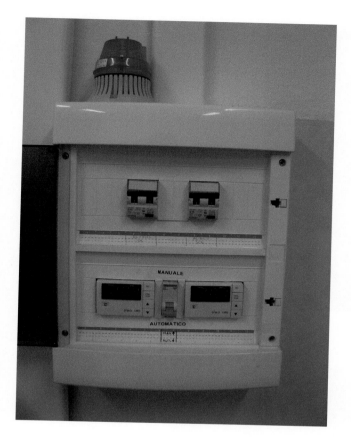

Figure 8.4 The electronic oxygen analyzer with alarm.

transferring to other containers, and the transport to other centers. These maneuvers must be performed in the briefest time possible in order to avoid the samples undergoing thermal injury, which can occur below the freezing point.

The time needed by different freezing devices to reach the critical air temperature of −7 °C during thawing is indicated:

Device	Temperature	Temperature	Time needed
Straw 0.25 ml	−196 °C	−7 °C	1.2 min
Straw 0.5 ml	−196 °C	−7 °C	2.2 min
Cryovial 0.5 ml	−196 °C	−7 °C	5.8 min

The thawing rate depends on the storage system used and on the quantity of liquid inside the device.

It is very important to put the straws (or other devices) of a patient inside a goblet (12 mm diameter) without perforating it. It is convenient to immerse the whole goblet into

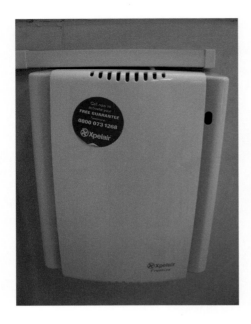

Figure 8.5 The internal air aspirator.

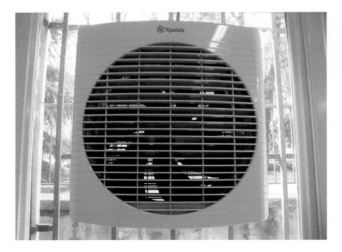

Figure 8.6 The ventilator (external air intake).

a small container of liquid nitrogen and insert the straws very rapidly inside it. Then the goblet is put inside the cryocontainer. This procedure allows the samples to remain always immersed; this is an important advantage when there is the need to move samples from one container to another or in the case of transfer to another center. The problem of correct transport is more critical in the case of vitrified samples because of the minimal volume.

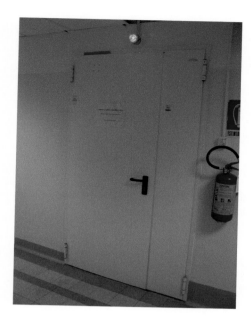

Figure 8.7 The external alarm.

To store biological samples belonging to infected patients, it is absolutely necessary to use high security straws and have different cryogenic containers for different pathologies.

The problem of cryopreserved oocyte transport to another center

More and more frequently, patients ask to transport samples from one center to another. In these cases, there is the problem of insuring the correct conservation of the samples to the point of destination. Precautions are taken to maintain the sample at a constant temperature. The goblets containing the samples must not be perforated, in order to avoid the outflow of the nitrogen when the samples are extracted from the cryocontainers. The goblet must be immediately inserted into the transport container. There are state-of-the-art transport containers: the Vapor shipper. They are internally provided with a porous substance which absorbs the liquid nitrogen and holds it, releasing the frigories in the form of vapor. They exist in various models of different dimensions and duration. The person in charge of carrying the biological samples comes to the center and takes the responsibility for appropriate transport to the destination. The transporter and the operator of the center where the samples are stored compile and sign documents attesting the identification of the samples and a receipt of delivery. Confirmation of delivery, by a fax from the receiving center, is mandatory to complete the procedure.

Database

Registration

The registration of the data is carried out both in paper registers and on the computer in order to assure operator, patient and sample identification.

Cryopreservation date, surname and name of the operator

Surname, name, date and place of birth of the patient

Surname, name, date and place of birth of the partner

Address, telephone number

Number of oocytes picked up and inseminated, insemination technique

Cryopreservation indication

Modality of the subdivision of the oocytes into the straws and the relative nuclear maturity

No. of the cryocontainer

No. of the canister

Goblet color

Jonc and goblet color

Pickup time

Cryopreservation time

Cryopreservation methodology

Solutions used, LOT Number and expiry date

At the moment of thawing, the following data are registered:

No. of the thawing cycle of the patient

Survived and degenerated oocytes

Residual cryopreserved oocytes

End time of thawing

The paper records and computers used to store data must be locked inside the cryobiological laboratory. The archive computer must be equipped with passwords for accessing sensitive data. It must be designed to back up the data.

Data updating

The data are updated for each new freezing and thawing. After each cycle of thawing, the number of remaining oocytes of the patient is recalculated.

Physician–embryologist cooperation for optimal management of the oocyte cryopreservation program

A description of the sequence of contacts which should exist between doctors and embryologists to ensure "safe" management of cryopreservation of oocytes is as follows.

For a program of cryopreservation of human oocytes to be safe and effective, it is essential that there is close collaboration between the doctors and the biologists. This is the only way to avoid misunderstandings and errors. The computerization of data in real time is essential for this purpose. The biologist immediately inserts the data about the freezing of gametes in the database so that the doctor can communicate the data to the patient with certainty. When the patient returns to program the thawing of the oocytes, the doctor fills out a report (see below) which is given to the biologist. The biologist ensures that the data are correct and tracks the samples. With this information, he/she returns the report to the doctor, who authorizes the patient to start therapy (or monitoring). The day before, the doctor tells the biologist the names of the patients whose oocytes will have to be thawed the following day. The biologist checks the programmed patients and the methodology used for cryopreservation to be sure to have ready the thawing solutions and the necessary materials. Any fact which deviates from normality must be communicated promptly.

Figure 10.1 shows the report for the traceability of the samples and the monitoring of the therapy.

SURNAME, NAME
DATE AND PLACE OF BIRTH

DATE O.P.U.   TELEPHONE NUMBER

☐ N° Frozen embryos _____

☐ N° Frozen oocytes _____

Date of report filling _____

M.D. signature _____

CHECK OF THE LAB.

DEWAR n° _____

Canister n° _____

Goblet color _____

Jonc color _____

Checking date _____

CONTROL   OK   ☐ yes ☐ no

Embryologist signature _____

NATURAL CYCLE

No therapy for the patient.

Last menstruation date_____ Signature _____

DATE	DAY CYCLE	ENDOMETRIUM	DX OVARY	SN OVARY	SIGNATURE

CLEARPLAN FROM _____ **DATE OF COLOR CHANGE** _____

TRANSFER DATE _____ **TIME** _____

ARTIFICIAL CYCLE Date of starting therapy ....../....../........

GnRH-a date _____ Last menstruation date_____Signature_____

DATE	☐ Estrogen _____ From _____	E2	END.	☐ Progestogen_____ From _____

TRANSFER DATE _____ **TIME** _____ **SEMEN SAMPLE date** _____ **time**_____

NOTES _____

Figure 10.1 Report for tracking samples and monitoring therapy.

Chapter

11

Costs

Cost of a slow freezing cycle

Instruments needed for a slow freezing cycle:

Instrument	Cost (euro)
Programmable freezer (Planer 360/1.79)	21 220.00
Electric pump for Planer	3 395.85
Tank Lab 30L (connect to the pressure pump)	1 393.60
Liquid supply	730.77
Dewar with 10 canisters	2 240.00
Self-pressurizing vessel	5 750.00
Pipette aid	275.00
Stereomicroscope	3 000.00
Total	**38 005.22**

Home-made solutions: a kit of 10 ml of each solution is prepared. A volume of 0.5 ml of the appropriate solution will be dispensed into each well. Each well accommodates one straw; thus, 10 ml of solution are enough for loading 20 straws. Considering that one, two, or three oocytes are loaded into each straw, the solutions are enough for freezing from 20 to 60 oocytes.

Materials needed for preparing 10 ml of each solution:

Material	Quantity	Cost (euro)
PBS	24 ml	0.48
1,2-propanediol	2.28 ml	0.1
Sucrose	0.684 g	0.1
DSS	6 ml	17.94
Sterile tips 1 ml	1	0.05
Sterile tips 10 ml	2	0.80
Falcon Tube 13 ml	9	2.88

(cont.)

Material	Quantity	Cost (euro)
Filter 0.2 μm	1	7.70
Syringe 10 ml	1	0.06
Total		**30.11**

Materials needed for a freezing cycle:

Material	Quantity	Cost (euro)
Sterile tips 1 ml	1	0.05
4 wells Nunclon	1 each straw	1.06
Pasteur pipette	1 each patient	0.2
Straw	1 for 1–3 oocytes	7.02
Jonc	1 each straw	3.42
Goblet 12 mm diameter	1 each patient	0.31
Metal stick	1 each patient	0.47
Liquid nitrogen	15L needed for one cycle	11.25
Total		**23.78**

Staff needed for a slow freezing cycle: one embryologist, one technician.

Cost of a thawing cycle

Homemade solutions: a kit of 10 ml of each solution is prepared. A volume of 0.5 ml of the appropriate solution will be dispensed into each well. Each well accommodates 1 straw; thus, 10 ml of the solution are enough for the thawing of 20 straws. Considering that one, two or three oocytes are loaded in each straw, the solutions are enough for freezing from 20 to 60 oocytes.

Materials needed for preparing 10 ml of each solution (one thawing kit):

Material	Quantity	Cost (euro)
PBS	36ml	0.6
1,2-propanediol	1.217ml	0.07
Sucrose	4.107 g (0.3 M)	0.6
DSS	8 ml	23.92
Sterile tips 1 ml	1	0.05
Sterile tips 10 ml	2	0.76

(*cont.*)

Material	Quantity	Cost (euro)
Flask 50 ml	2	1.6
Falcon Tube 13 ml	12	3.8
Filter 0.2 μm	1	7.74
Syringe 10 ml	1	0.06
Total		**39.20**

Materials needed for a thawing cycle:

Material	Quantity	Cost (euro)
4 wells Nunclon	1 for straw + 1 for culture	2.12
Pasteur pipette	1 for patient	0.14
Sterile tips 1 ml	1 for patient	0.11
Liquid nitrogen	0.5 L	0.375
Thermometer	1	12.6
Sterile surgical type scissors	1	20.00
Insulin type syringe with silicone adaptor	1 each straw	1.0
Total		**36.35**

Staff needed for a thawing cycle: one embryologist.

Cost of a vitrification cycle

Costs of instruments needed for vitrification:

Instrument	Cost (euro)
Pipette aid	275.00
Gilson pipette 1–20 μl	198.00
Pipette for denuding capillary	300.00
Aspiration pump (only for Cryotop)	1 000.00
System for liquid nitrogen filtration (only for Cryotop)	148.00
Stereomicroscope	3 000.00
Adjustable heat stage	3 500.00
Thermal sealer (HSV) or Impulse sealer (Cryotip)	2 000.00 or 200.00
Total	**7 273.00** (price calculated without the instruments in italics)

Homemade solutions: the volume of wash solution (WS) and equilibration solution (ES) used is very low (70 μl each), while 0.5 ml of vitrification solution (VS) are needed for each device. Thus, 10 ml of VS are enough for 20 devices (each of which can hold one, two or three oocytes), while WS and ES will be in excess. It is possible to prepare a smaller volume of WS and ES to save materials (keep in mind that WS can also be used for warming).

Materials needed for preparing 10 ml of each solution (one vitrification kit):

Material	Quantity	Cost (euro)
Ethylene glycol (EG)	2.25 ml	0.09
Dimethyl sulfoxide (DMSO)	2.25 ml	2.50
Sucrose	1.7115 g	4.67
Ham's F10	36 ml	0.72
DSS	6 ml	17.94
Falcon Tube 13 ml	6	1.92
Filter 0.2 μm	1	7.70
Syringe 10 ml	1	0.06
Sterile tips 1 ml	2	0.10
Sterile tips 10 ml	2	0.76
Cryovial	30 cryovials for kit	15.00
Total		**51.46**

Materials needed for a vitrification cycle:

Material	Quantity	Cost (euro)
4 wells Nunclon	2	2.12
Sterile tips	3 for device	0.33
Denuding capillary	1 for device	5.60
Storing device (HSV)	1	12.00
Storing device (Cryotip)	1	33.40
Storing device (Cryotop)	1	8.00
Omnipore sterile filter (only for Cryotop)	1 each patient	3.00
Liquid nitrogen	0.5–3.0 L	0.37 (or 2.25 considering filtration)
Goblet 12 mm diameter	1 each patient	1.08
Metal stick		0.47
Total		**9.97** (this price is calculated without the materials in italics)

Staff needed for a vitrification cycle: one embryologist.

Cost of a warming cycle

Homemade solutions: for each device that has to be warmed, 0.8 ml of thawing solution (TS) and diluent solution (DS) and 1.0 ml of WS are needed. Regarding the use of WS, 10 ml of solution are enough to warm about 20 devices. It is possible to prepare a smaller volume of TS and DS to save materials.

Materials needed for preparing 10 ml of each solution (one warming kit):

Material	Quantity	Cost (euro)
Sucrose	5.134 g	0.72
Ham's F10	24 ml	0.48
DSS	6 ml	17.94
Falcon Tube 13 ml	6	1.92
Filter 0.2 μm	1	7.70
Syringe 10 ml	1	0.06
Cryovial	30 for kit	15.00
Total		**43.82**

Materials needed for a warming cycle:

Material	Quantity	Cost (euro)
4 wells Nunclon	2 for device + 1 for culture	3.2
1 ml sterile tip	1 for patient	0.05
Liquid nitrogen	0.5 L	0.375
Denuding pipette	1 for device	5.5
Total		**9.13**

Staff needed for a warming cycle: one embryologist.

Comparison between slow freezing and vitrification

Methodology	Cost of instruments	Staff
Slow freezing	38 005.47 euro	1 embryologist + 1 technician
Vitrification	7 273.00 euro	1 embryologist

Methodology	Cost of a kit of 10 ml of each solution (in euro)	Cost of materials needed for a cycle (in euro)
Slow freezing	30.11	23.78
Rapid thawing	39.20	36.34
TOTAL	**69.31**	**60.12**
Vitrification	51.46	9.97**
Warming	43.82	9.13
TOTAL	**95.28**	**19.10**

** The price of the device has to be added to this cost: HSV = 12 euro; Cryotip = 33.4 euro; Cryotop = 8 euro; Omnipore filter = 3 euro.

Staff

Chapter

12

The number of people needed in the laboratory for the proper carrying out of all projected operations is one biologist and one technician, who are 100% involved in the program of oocyte cryopreservation. Periodically, these people must switch with other colleagues. At least five properly educated people who can alternate in filling up the liquid nitrogen are necessary.

Tricks and secrets of oocyte cryopreservation

Preparation of cryopreservation solutions

When the sucrose is contained in a solution find an indication like this: *0.342 g SUCROSE + 4 ml PBS + 1.14 ml PROH and solubilize; make up to a volume of 7 ml with PBS.* This means that you have first to weigh the sucrose, then add a volume of PBS and PROH and solubilize the sucrose. Only after the solubilization of the sucrose, can you add PBS until the final volume is reached. Because the sucrose "takes up space inside the tube," only by solubilizing it first, are you sure to reach the correct molarity of the final solution.

Cryopreservation solutions have to be filtered starting from the least concentrated to higher concentrated ones. They have to be stored at $+4\,^{\circ}C$, and can be stored and utilized for 60 days from the day of preparation if they are stored correctly. The date of preparation is utilized as the LOT Number. They are listed in an informatized inventory.

Freezing

The time required for incubation into freezing solutions and loading of the samples varies from 20 minutes to 35 minutes. This time can change with a variation in the number of oocytes that must be frozen in that cycle. Freezing an excessive number of oocytes per cycle is not recommended so that these times are not exceeded.

Move the sample from one solution to the other by keeping it in a small quantity of the solution and releasing it into the next solution. In this way the passage will be less shocking.

Leave the samples for at least 10 minutes at $-150\,^{\circ}C$ to reach a good equilibration before taking them out of the machine for storing. Store the samples in a goblet of 12 mm diameter without making holes in the plastic. In this way, when the goblet is extracted, the samples continue to stay immersed in the liquid nitrogen and are less likely to be submitted to temperature changes. It is very important to place the straws or devices for each patient into a goblet without perforating it.

Thawing

The first two steps of the procedure are more critical: 30 seconds at air and 40 seconds in a $30\,^{\circ}C$ water-bath. You have to be very precise regarding these times.

The passages from one solution to another are carried out by collecting the oocyte in a small quantity of the solution that they are in and releasing them into the next solution. This makes the transition from one molarity to another less shocking.

An oocyte which truly survives after cryopreservation must appear morphologically the same as a fresh oocyte at the end of the thawing procedure. When the cytoplasm is dark or transparent, the perivitelline space (PVS) is absent because of the oolemma rupture and the oocyte has to be discarded.

The definition of survival does not include the capacity to be fertilized. However, if the subsequent fertilization rate is strongly impaired, a more accurate assessment of survival is advised. It is not uncommon to find that an oocyte survives with the first polar body degenerated at the end of the procedure. This oocyte can be used for insemination. It is important to register this finding to make a correct interpretation of subsequent fertilization.

The embryo check is carried out on the second to third day. It is important to point out that the cleavage of embryos so obtained from thawed oocytes is slightly lower than that of fresh embryos; thus, four-cell embryos are frequently found on the third day.

Vitrification

It is very important to keep out the culture oil at the beginning of the procedure. This will facilitate the next steps. Furthermore, it is very important to keep in mind the starting oocyte's morphology and the PVS size. This will let you know the moment to stop the incubation in ES3.

Minimum volume

This concept (Kuwayama, 2007) means that the sample has to be loaded on the device with the smallest possible volume of solution. This could be done by loading the sample in a small volume and leaving it at the tip of the denuding pipette. Then, the excess volume has to be taken out by aspirating it with the denuding pipette until the sample is covered only by a thin layer of liquid. This concept is very important, because the smaller the volume, the quicker will be the vitrification process and the greater its efficacy.

References

Abir R, Fisch B, Nahum R, *et al.* Turner's syndrome and fertility: current status and possible putative prospects. *Hum Reprod Update* 2001;7:603–10.

Aigner S, Van der Elst J, Siebzehnrubl E, *et al.* The influence of slow and ultra-rapid freezing on the organization of the meiotic spindle in the mouse oocyte. *Hum Reprod* 1992;7:857–64.

Al-Hasani S, Diedrich K. Oocyte storage. In: Grudzinskas JG, Yovich JL, editors. Gametes-The Oocyte. Cambridge: Cambridge University Press;1995, 376–95.

Al-Hasani S, Diedrich K, van der Ven H, Krebs D. Initial results of the cryopreservation of human oocytes. *Geburthshilfe Franuehilkild* 1986;6:643–4.

Al-Hasani S, Diedrich K, van der Ven H, *et al.* Cryopreservation of human oocytes. *Hum Reprod* 1987;2:695–700.

Allan J. Re: case report: pregnancy from intracytoplasmic injection of a frozen-thawed oocyte. *Aust N Z J Obstet Gynaecol* 2004;44(6):588.

Antinori S, Dani G, Selman HA, *et al.* Pregnancies after sperm injection into cryopreserved human oocytes. *Hum Reprod* 1998;13:157–8.

Antinori M, Licata E, Dani G, *et al.* Cryotop vitrification of human oocytes results in high survival rate and healthy deliveries. *Reprod Biomed Online* 2007;14:72–9.

Asahina E. Intracellular freezing and frost resistance in egg-cells of the sea urchin. *Nature* 1961;191:1263–5.

Aso K, Koto S, Higuchi A, *et al.* Serum FSH level below 10 mIU/mL at twelve years old is an index of spontaneous and cyclical menstruation in Turner syndrome. *Endocrine J* 2010;57(10):909–13.

Ata B, Chian RC, Tan SL. Cryopreservation of oocytes and embryos for fertility preservation for female cancer patients. *Best Pract Res Clin Obstet Gynaecol* 2010;24:101–12.

Attar E, Berkman S, Topuz S, *et al.* Evolutive peritoneal disease after conservative management and the use of infertility drugs in a patient with stage IIIC borderline micro-papillary serous carcinoma (MPSC) of the ovary: case report. *Hum Reprod* 2004;19(6):1472–5.

Azambuja R, Badalotti M, Teloken C, Michelon J, Petracco A. Successful birth after injection of frozen human oocytes with frozen epididymal spermatozoa. *Reprod Biomed Online* 2005;11:449–51.

Azambuja R, Petracco A, Okada L, *et al.* Experience of freezing human oocytes using sodium-depleted media. *Reprod Biomed Online* 2011;22(1):83–7.

Azim A, Oktay K. Letrozole for ovulation induction and fertility preservation by embryo cryopreservation in young women with endometrial carcinoma. *Fertil Steril* 2007;88(3):657–64.

Azim A, Ferrando MC, Lostritto K, Oktay K. Relative potencies of anastrozole and letrozole to suppress estradiol in breast cancer patients undergoing ovarian stimulation before in vitro fertilization. *J Clin Endocrinol Metab* 2007a;92(6):2197–200.

Azim A, Costantini-Ferrando M, Oktay K. Safety of fertility preservation by ovarian stimulation with letrozole and gonadotropins in patients with breast cancer: a prospective controlled study. *J Clin Oncol* 2008;26(16):2630–5.

Bahadur G. Fertility issues for cancer patients. *Mol Cell Endocrinol* 2000;169(1–2): 117–22.

Baka SG, Toth TL, Veeck LL, *et al.* Evaluation of the spindle apparatus of in-vitro matured human oocytes following cryopreservation. *Hum Reprod* 1995; 10(7):1816–20.

Bakalov V, Shawker T, Ceniceros I, Bondy CA. Uterine development in Turner syndrome. *J Pediatr* 2007;**151**(5):528–31.

Balakier H, Bouman D, Sojecki A, *et al.* Morphological and cytogenetic analysis of human giant oocytes and giant embryos. *Hum Reprod* 2002;**17**:2394–401.

Balash J, Gratacós E. Delayed childbearing: effects on fertility and the outcome of pregnancy. *Fetal Diagn Ther* 2011;**29**:263–73.

Bankowski B, Lyverly AD, Faden RR, Wallach EE. The social implications of embryo cryopreservation. *Fertil Steril* 2005;**4**:823–32.

Barritt J, Luna M, Duke M, *et al.* Report of four donor-recipient oocyte cryopreservation cycles resulting in high pregnancy and implantation. *Fertil Steril* 2007;**87**:189.e13–17.

Bernard A, Fuller BJ. Cryopreservation of human oocytes: a review of current problems and perspectives. *Hum Reprod Update* 1996;**2**:193–207.

Bernard A, Imoedembe DA, Shaw RW, Fuller B. Effects of cryprotectants on human oocytes. *Lancet* 1985;**1**:632–3.

Bianchi V, Coticchio G, Fava L, Flamigni C, Borini A. Meiotic spindle imaging in human oocytes frozen with a slow freezing procedure involving high sucrose concentration. *Hum Reprod* 2005;**20**:1078–83.

Bianchi V, Coticchio G, Distratis V, *et al.* Differential sucrose concentration during dehydration (0.2 mol/l) and rehydration (0.3 mol/l) increases the implantation rate of frozen human oocytes. *Reprod Biomed Online* 2007;**14**:64–71.

Bianchi V, Lappi M, Bonu MA, Borini A. Oocyte slow freezing using a 0.2–0.3 M sucrose concentration protocol: is it really the time to trash the cryopreservation machine? *Fertil Steril* 2012;**97**(5):1101–7.

Birkebaek N, Crüger D, Hansen J. Fertility and pregnancy outcome in Danish women with Turner syndrome. *Clin Genet* 2002;**61**:34–9.

Bodri D, Vernaeve V, Figueras F, *et al.* Oocyte donation in patients with Turner's syndrome: a successful technique but with an accompanying high risk of hypertensive disorders during pregnancy. *Hum Reprod* 2006;**21**:829–32.

Boiso I, Mati M, Santalo J, *et al.* A confocal microscopy analysis of the spindle and chromosome configurations of human oocytes cryopreserved at the germinal vesicle and metaphase II stage. *Hum Reprod* 2002;**17**:1885–91.

Boissonnas CC, Davy C, Bornes M, *et al.* Careful cardiovascular screening and follow-up of women with Turner syndrome before and during pregnancy is necessary to prevent maternal mortality. *Fertil Steril* 2009;**91**(3):929.e5–7.

Boldt J, Cline D, McLaughlin D. Human oocyte cryopreservation as an adjunct to IVF-embryo transfer cycles. *Hum Reprod* 2003;**18**:1250–5.

Boldt J, Tidswell N, Sayers A, Kilani R, Cline D. Human oocyte cryopreservation: 5-year experience with a sodium-depleted slow freezing method. *Reprod Biomed Online* 2006;**13**:96–100.

Bondy CA. Turner Syndrome Study Group. Care of girls and women with Turner syndrome: a guideline of the Turner Syndrome Study Group. *J Clin Endocrinol Metab* 2007;**92**:10–25.

Borgstrom B, Hreinsson J, Rasmussen C, *et al.* Fertility preservation in girls with Turner syndrome: prognostic signs of the presence of ovarian follicles. *J Clin Endocrinol Metab* 2009;**94**(1):74–80.

Borini A, Bafaro MG, Bonu MA, *et al.* Pregnancies after oocyte freezing and thawing, preliminary data. *Hum Reprod* 1998;**13**:124–5.

Borini A, Bonu MA, Coticchio G, *et al.* Pregnancies and births after oocyte cryopreservation. *Fertil Steril* 2004;**82**(3):601–5.

Borini A, Lagalla C, Bonu MA, *et al.* Cumulative pregnancy rates resulting from the use of fresh and frozen oocytes: 7 years' experience. *Reprod Biomed Online* 2006a; **12**:481–6.

Borini A, Sciajno R, Bianchi V, *et al.* Clinical outcome of oocyte cryopreservation after slow cooling with a protocol utilizing a high sucrose concentration. *Hum Reprod* 2006b;**21**:512–17.

Borini A, Bianchi V, Bonu MA, *et al.* Evidence-based clinical outcome of oocyte slow cooling. *Reprod Biomed Online* 2007a;**15**:175–81.

Borini A, Cattoli M, Mazzone S, *et al.* Survey of 105 babies born after slow cooling oocyte cryopreservation. *Fertil Steril* 2007b;**88**:S13.

Borini A, Levi Setti PE, Anserini P, *et al.* Multicenter observational study on slow-cooling oocyte cryopreservation: clinical outcome. *Fertil Steril* 2010;**94**(5):1662–8.

Brugger EC. "Other selves": moral and legal proposals regarding the personhood of cryopreserved human embryos. *Theor Med Bioeth* 2009;**30**:105–29.

Bryman I, Sylvén L, Berntorp K, *et al.* Pregnancy rate and outcome in Swedish women with Turner syndrome. *Fertil Steril* 2011;**95**(8):2507–10.

Burks JL. Morphologic evaluation of frozen rabbit and human ova. *Fertil Steril* 1965;**16**:638–41.

Cabanes L, Chalas C, Christin-Maitre S, *et al.* Turner syndrome and pregnancy: clinical practice. Recommendations for the management of patients with Turner syndrome before and during pregnancy. *Eur J Obstet Gynecol Reprod Biol* 2010;**152**:18–24.

Cao YX, Chian RC. Fertility preservation with immature and in vitro matured oocytes. *Semin Reprod Med* 2009;**27**(6):456–64.

Cha KY, Koo JJ, Ko JJ, *et al.* Pregnancy after in vitro fertilization of human follicular oocytes collected from nonstimulated cycles, their culture in vitro and their transfer in donor oocyte program. *Fertil Steril* 1991;**55**:109–13.

Chamayou S, Alecci C, Ragolia C, *et al.* Comparison of in-vitro outcomes from cryopreserved oocytes and sibling fresh oocytes. *Reprod Biomed Online* 2006;**12**:730–6.

Chang CC. Two successful pregnancies obtained following oocyte vitrification and embryo re-vitrification. *Reprod BioMed Online* 2008;**16**(3):346–9.

Chang CC, Shapiro DB, Bernal DP, *et al.* Human oocyte vitrification: in-vivo and in-vitro maturation outcomes. *Reprod Biomed Online* 2008a;**17**(5):684–8.

Chang MC. Probability of normal development after transplantation of fertilized rabbit ova

stored at different temperatures. *Proc Soc Exp Biol Med* 1948a;**161**:978.

Chang MC. Transplantation of fertilized rabbit ova: the effect on viability of age, in vitro storage period, and storage temperature. *Nature* 1948b;**159**:602.

Chang MC. Storage of unfertilized rabbit ova: subsequent fertilization and the probability of normal development. *Nature* 1953;**172**:353–4.

Chen C. Pregnancy after human oocyte cryopreservation. *Lancet* 1986;**1**:884–6.

Chen C. Pregnancies after human oocyte cryopreservation. *Ann N Y Acad Sci* 1988;**541**:541–9.

Chen SU, Lien YR, Tsai YY, *et al.* Successful pregnancy occurred from slowly freezing human oocytes using the regime of 1.5 mol/l 1,2 propanediol with 0.3 mol/l sucrose. *Hum Reprod* 2002;**17**:1412–13.

Chen SU, Lien YR, Chen HF, *et al.* Observational clinical follow-up of oocyte cryopreservation using a slow freezing method with 1,2-propanediol plus sucrose followed by ICSI. *Hum Reprod* 2005;**20**:1975–80.

Chen ZJ, Li M, Li Y, *et al.* Effects of sucrose concentration on the developmental potential of human frozen-thawed oocytes at different stages of maturity. *Hum Reprod* 2004;**19**(10):2345–9.

Chia C, Chan W, Quah E, Cheng L. Triploid pregnancy after ICSI of frozen testicular spermatozoa into cryopreserved human oocytes. Case report. *Hum Reprod* 2000;**15**:1962–4.

Chian RC, Son WY, Huang JY, *et al.* High survival rates and pregnancies of human oocytes following vitrification: preliminary report. *Fertil Steril* 2005;**84**:S36.

Chian RC, Huang JY, Tan SL, *et al.* Obstetrics and perinatal outcome in 200 infants conceived from vitrified oocytes. *Reprod Biomed Online* 2008;**16**(5):608–10.

Chian RC, Gilbert L, Huang JYJ, *et al.* Live birth after vitrification of in vitro matured human oocytes. *Fertil Steril* 2009;**91**(2):372–6.

Choung CJ. Effects of cryopreservation on the viability and fertilizability of unfertilized hamster oocytes. *Am J Obstet Gynecol* 1986;**155**(6):1240–5.

Ciotti PM, Notarangelo L, Morrselli-Labate AM, *et al.* First polar body morphology is not related to embryo quality or pregnancy rate. *Hum Reprod* 2004;**19**(10):2334–9.

Ciotti PM, Porcu E, Notarangelo L, *et al.* Meiotic spindle recovery is faster in vitrification of human oocytes compared to slow freezing. *Fertil Steril* 2009;**91**(6):2399–407.

Cobo A, Rubio C, Gerli S, *et al.* Use of fluorescence in situ hybridization to assess the chromosomal status of embryos obtained from cryopreserved oocytes. *Fertil Steril* 2001;**75**:354–60.

Cobo A, Bellver J, Domingo J, *et al.* New options in assisted reproduction technology: the Cryotop method of oocyte vitrification. *Reprod Biomed Online* 2008a;**17**:68–72.

Cobo A, Domingo J, Perez S, *et al.* Vitrification: an effective new approach to oocyte banking and preserving fertility in cancer patients. *Clin Transl Oncol* 2008b;**10**:268–73.

Cobo A, Kuwayama M, Perez S, *et al.* Comparison of concomitant outcome achieved with fresh and cryopreserved donor oocytes vitrified by the Cryotop method. *Fertil Steril* 2008c;**89**:1657–64.

Cobo A, Perez S, Zulategui J, *et al.* Effect of different cryopreservation protocols on the metaphase II spindle in human oocytes. *Reprod Biomed Online* 2008d;**17**:350–9.

Committee on Gynecologic Practice of American College of Obstetricians and Gynecologists; Practice Committee of American Society for Reproductive Medicine. Age-related fertility decline: a committee opinion. *Fertil Steril* 2008;**90**(5 suppl):S154–5.

Coticchio G, De Santis L, Rossi G, *et al.* Sucrose concentration influences the rate of human oocytes with normal spindle and chromosome configurations after slow-cooling cryopreservation. *Hum Reprod* 2006;**21**(7):1771–6.

Critser JK. Cryopreservation of hamster oocytes: effects of vitrification or freezing on human sperm penetration of zona-free hamster oocytes. *Fertil Steril* 1986;**46**(2):277–84.

De Geyter M, Steimann S, Holzgreve W, De Geyter C. First delivery of healthy offspring after freezing and thawing of oocytes in Switzerland. *Swiss Med Wkly* 2007;**137**:443–7.

Demirtas E, Elizur SE, Holzer H, *et al.* Immature oocyte retrieval in the luteal phase to preserve fertility in women with cancer facing imminent gonadotoxic therapy: it is worth a try. *Reprod Biomed Online* 2008;**17**:520–3.

De Santis L, Cino I, Rabellotti E, *et al.* Oocyte cryopreservation: clinical outcome of slow-cooling protocols differing in sucrose concentration. *Reprod Biomed Online* 2006;**14**:57–63.

Diedrich K, Al-Hasani S, van der Ver H, Krebs D. Successful in vitro fertilization of frozen-thawed rabbit and human oocytes. *Ann N Y Acad Sci* 1988;**541**:562–71.

Ding J, Rana N, Dmowski WP. Successful pregnancies after oocyte cryopreservation with slow-freezing method: a report of 3 cases. *J Reprod Med* 2008;**53**(10):813–20.

Doerr HG, Bettendorf M, Hauffa BP, *et al.* Uterine size in women with Turner syndrome after induction of puberty with estrogens and long-term growth hormone therapy: results of the German IGLU Follow-up Study 2001. *Hum Reprod* 2005;**20**:1418–21.

Doherty L, Pal L. Reproductive banking and older women. *Maturitas* 2011;**70**(1):3–4.

Donnez J, Dolmans M, Demylle D, *et al.* Livebirth after orthotopic transplantation of cryopreserved ovarian tissue. *Lancet* 2004;**364**:1405–10.

Dumoulin JCM, Bergers-Janssen JM, Pieters MH, *et al.* The protective effect of polymers in the cryopreservation of human and mouse zonae pellucidae and embryos. *Fertil Steril* 1994;**62**:793–8.

Ebner T, Moser M, Yaman C, *et al.* Elective transfer of embryos selected on the basis of first polar body morphology is associated with increased rates of implantation and pregnancy. *Fertil Steril* 1999;**72**:599–603.

Ebner T, Moser M, Sommergruber C, *et al.* First polar body morphology and blastocyst formation rate in ICSI patients. *Hum Reprod* 2002;**17**:2415–18.

Edwards RG. Maturation in vitro of human ovarian oocytes. *Lancet* 1965;**2**:926–9.

Eichenlaub-Ritter U, Schmiady H, Kentenich H, *et al.* Recurrent failure in polar body formation and premature chromosome condensation in oocytes from a human patient: indicators of asynchrony in nuclear and cytoplasmic maturation *Hum Reprod* 1995;**10**:2343–9.

Elizur SE, Beiner ME, Korach J, *et al.* Outcome of in vitro fertilization treatment in infertile women conservatively treated for endometrial adenocarcinoma. *Fertil Steril* 2007;**88**(6):1562–7.

El-Shawarby SA, Sharif AF, Conway G, Serhal P, Davies M. Oocyte cryopreservation after controlled ovarian hyperstimulation in mosaic Turner syndrome: another fertility preservation option in a dedicated UK clinic. *BJOG* 2010;**117**(2):234–7.

Ezcurra D, Rangnow J, Craig M, Schertz J. The Human Oocyte Preservation Experience (HOPE) a phase IV, prospective, multicenter, observational oocyte cryopreservation registry. *Reprod Biol Endocrinol* 2009;**7**:53.

Fabbri R, Porcu E, Marsella T, *et al.* Human oocyte cryopreservation: new perspectives regarding oocyte survival. *Hum Reprod* 2001;**16**:411–16.

Fasouliotis SJ, Davis O, Schattman G, *et al.* Safety and efficacy of infertility treatment after conservative management of borderline ovarian tumors: a preliminary report. *Fertil Steril* 2004;**82**(3):568–72.

Fortin A, Morice P, Thoury A, *et al.* Impact of infertility drugs after treatment of borderline ovarian tumors: results of a retrospective multicenter study. *Fertil Steril* 2007;**87**(3):591–6.

Fosas N, Marina F, Torres PJ, *et al.* The births of five Spanish babies from cryopreserved donated oocytes. *Hum Reprod* 2003;**18**:1417–21.

Foudila T, Soderstrom-Anttila V, Hovatta O. Turner's syndrome and pregnancies after oocyte donation. *Hum Reprod* 1999;**14**:532–5.

Funaki K, Mikamo K. Giant diploid oocytes as a cause of digynic triploidy in mammals. *Cytogenet Cell Genet* 1980;**28**:158–68.

Gardner DK, Courtney BS, Rienzi L, Katz-Jaffe M, Larman MG. Analysis of oocyte physiology to improve cryopreservation procedures. *Theriogenology* 2007;**67**:64–72.

George MA, Pickering SJ, Braude PR, Johnson MH. The distribution of a- and g-tubulin in fresh and aged mouse and human oocytes

exposed to cryoprotectant. *Mol Hum Reprod* 1996;**2**:445–56.

Glenister PH, Wood MJ, Kirby C, Whittingham DG. Incidence of chromosome anomalies in first-cleavage mouse embryos obtained from frozen-thawed oocytes fertilized in vitro. *Gamete Res* 1987;**16**:205–16.

Goodwin PJ, Ennis M, Pritchard KI, Trudeau M, Hood N. Risk of menopause during the first year after breast cancer. *J Clin Oncol* 1999;**17**(8):2365–70.

Gook DA, Edgar DH. Human oocyte cryopreservation. *Hum Reprod Update* 2007;**13**:591–605.

Gook D, Osborn SM, Johnston WI. Cryopreservation of mouse and human oocytes using 1,2 propanediol and the configuration of the meiotic spindle. *Hum Reprod* 1993;**8**:1101–9.

Gook D, Osborn SM, Bourne H, Johnston WI. Fertilization of human oocytes following cryopreservation; normal karyotypes and absence of stray chromosomes. *Hum Reprod* 1994;**9**:684–91.

Gook DA, Osborn SM, Johnston WI. Parthenogenetic activation of human oocytes following cryopreservation using 1,2-propanediol. *Hum Reprod* 1995a;**10**:654–8.

Gook D, Schiewe MC, Osborn SM, *et al.* Intracytoplasmic sperm injection and embryo development of human oocytes cryopreserved using 1,2-propanediol. *Hum Reprod* 1995b;**10**:2637–41.

Gook DA, Osborn SM, Archer J, Edgar DH, McBain J. Follicle development following cryopreservation of human ovarian tissue. *Eur J Obstet Gynecol Reprod Biol* 2004;**113** (Suppl 1):S60–2.

Gook DA, Hale L, Edgar DH. Live birth following transfer of a cryopreserved embryo generated from a cryopreserved oocyte and a cryopreserved sperm: case report. *J Assist Reprod Genet* 2007a;**24**:43–5.

Goold I, Savulescu J. In favour of freezing eggs for non-medical reasons. *Bioethics* 2009;**23** (1):47–58

Gosden RG. Gonadal tissue cryopreservation and transplantation. *Reprod Biomed Online* 2002;**4**(Suppl 1):64–7.

References

Hadnott TN, Gould HN, Gharib AM, Bondy CA. Outcomes of spontaneous and assisted pregnancies in Turner syndrome: the US National Institute of Health experience. *Fertil Steril* 2011;**95**(7):2251–6.

Hagen CP, Aksglaede L, Sørensen K, *et al.* Serum levels of anti-Mullerian hormone as a marker of ovarian function in 926 healthy females from birth to adulthood and in 172 Turner syndrome patients. *J Clin Endocrinol Metab* 2010;**95**:5003–10.

Hjerrild BE, Mortensen KH, Gravholt CH. Turner syndrome and clinical treatment. *Br Med Bull* 2008;**86**:77–93.

Hoffman JS, Laird L, Benadiva C, Dreiss R. In vitro fertilization following conservative management of stage 3 serous borderline tumor of the ovary. *Gynecol Oncol* 1999;**74**:515–18.

Hoffman DI, Zellman GL, Fair CC, *et al.* Cryopreserved embryos in the United States and their availability for research. *Fertil Steril* 2003;**79**:1063–9.

Hong SW, Chung HM, Lim JM, *et al.* Improved human oocyte development after vitrification: a comparison of thawing methods. *Fertil Steril* 1999;**72**(1):142–6.

Hreinsson JG, Otala M, Fridström M, *et al.* Follicles are found in the ovaries of adolescent girls with Turner's syndrome. *J Clin Endocrinol Metab* 2002;**87**:3618–23.

Huang JY, Buckett WM, Gilbert L, Tan SL, Chian RC. Retrieval of immature oocytes followed by in vitro maturation and vitrification: a case report on a new strategy of fertility preservation in women with borderline ovarian malignancy. *Gynecol Oncol* 2007a;**105**(2):542–4.

Huang JY, Chen HY, Park JY, Tan SL, Chian RC. Comparison of spindle and chromosome configuration in in vitro- and in vivo-matured mouse oocytes after vitrification. *Fertil Steril* 2007b;**90**(4 suppl):1424–32.

Huang JYJ, Tulandi T, Holzer H, *et al.* Cryopreservation of ovarian tissue and in vitro matured oocytes in a female with mosaic Turner syndrome: case Report. *Hum Reprod* 2008a;**23**(2):336–9

Huang JY, Tulandi T, Holzer H, Tan SL, Chian RC. Combining ovarian tissue cryobanking with retrieval of immature oocytes followed by in vitro maturation and vitrification: an additional strategy of fertility preservation. *Fertil Steril* 2008b;**89**(3):567–72.

Huttelova R, Becvarova V, Brachtlova T. More successful oocyte freezing. *J Assist Reprod Genet* 2003;**20**(8):293.

Joly C, Bchini O, Boulekbache H, Testart J, Maro B. Effects of 1,2-propanediol on the cytoskeletal organisation of the mouse oocyte. *Hum Reprod* 1992;**3**:374–8.

Kahraman S, Yakin K, Donmez E, *et al.* Relationship between granular cytoplasm of oocytes and pregnancy outcome following intracytoplasmic sperm injection. *Hum Reprod* 2000;**15**:2390–3.

Katayama KP, Stehlik J, Kuwayama M, *et al.* High survival rate of vitrified human oocytes results in clinical pregnancy. *Fertil Steril* 2003;**80**:223–4.

Kazem R, Thompson LA, Srikantharajah A, *et al.* Cryopreservation of human oocytes and fertilization by two techniques: in-vitro fertilization and intracytoplasmic sperm injection. *Hum Reprod* 1995;**10**:2650–4.

Keefe D, Liu L, Wang W, Silva C. Imaging meiotic spindles by polarization light microscopy: principles and applications to IVF. *Reprod Biomed Online* 2003;**4**:24–9.

Khastgir G, Abdalla H, Thomas A, *et al.* Oocyte donation in Turner's syndrome: an analysis of the factors affecting the outcome. *Hum Reprod* 1997;**12**(2):279–85.

Kim TJ, Hong SW, Park SE, Cha KY. Pregnancy after vitrification of human oocytes and blastocysts using same cryoprotectant solution, ethylene glycol and sucrose. *Fertil Steril* 2003;**80**:S143.

Kim T, Hong S, Cha K. Pregnancies from cryopreserved oocytes using vitrification protocol. *Fertil Steril* 2005;**84**(Suppl 1):S179.

King CR, Magenis E, Bennett S. Pregnancy and the Turner syndrome. *Obstet Gynecol* 1978;**52**(5):617–24.

Klock SC, Sheinin S, Kazer RR. The disposition of unused frozen embryos. *N Engl J Med* 2001;**345**:69–70.

Kola I, Kirby C, Shaw J, Davey A, Trounson A. Vitrification of mouse oocytes results in aneuploid zygotes and malformed fetuses. *Teratology* 1988;**38**:467–74.

Konc J, Kanyo K, Cseh S. Does oocyte cryopreservation have a future in Hungary? *Reprod Biomed Online* 2007;**14**:11–13.

Konc J, Kanyo K, Varga E, Kriston R, Cseh S. Oocyte cryopreservation: the birth of the first Hungarian babies from frozen oocytes. *J Assist Reprod Genet* 2008a;**25**:349–52.

Konc J, Kanyo K, Varga E, Kriston R, Cseh S. Births resulting from oocyte cryopreservation using a slow freezing protocol with propanediol and sucrose. *Syst Biol Reprod Med* 2008b;**54**(4–5):205–10.

Kuleshova L, Gianaroli L, Magli C, *et al.* Birth following vitrification of a small number of human oocytes: case report. *Hum Reprod* 1999;**14**:3077–9.

Kuwayama M. Highly efficient vitrification for cryopreservation of human oocytes and embryos: the Cryotop method. *Theriogenology* 2007;**67**(1):73–80.

Kuwayama M, Vajta G, Kato O, Leibo SP. Highly efficient vitrification method for cryopreservation of human oocytes. *Reprod Biomed Online* 2005;**11**:300–8.

Kyono K, Fuchinoue K, Yagi A, *et al.* Successful pregnancy and delivery after transfer of a single blastocyst derived from a vitrified mature human oocyte. *Fertil Steril* 2005;**84**:1017.

Larman MG, Sheehan CB, Gardner DK. Calcium free vitrification reduces cryoprotectant-induced zona pellucida hardening and increases fertilization rates in mouse oocytes. *Reproduction* 2006;**131**:53–61

Larman MG, Katz-Jaffe MG, Sheehan CB, Gardner DK. 1,2-propanediol and the type of cryopreservation procedure adversely affect mouse oocyte physiology. *Hum Reprod* 2007a;**22**:250–9

Larman MG, Minasi MG, Rienzi L, Gardner DK. Maintenance of the meiotic spindle during vitrification in human and mouse oocytes. *Reprod Biomed Online* 2007b;**15**:692–700.

La Sala GB, Vicoli A, Villani MT, *et al.* Outcome of 518 salvage oocyte-cryopreservation cycles performed as a routine procedure in an in vitro fertilization program. *Fertil Steril* 2006;**86**:1423–7.

Lassalle B, Testart J, Renard JP. Human embryo features that influence the success of cryopreservation with the use of 1,2 propanediol. *Fertil Steril* 1985;**44**:645–51.

Lau NM, Huang JY, MacDonald S, *et al.* Feasibility of fertility preservation in young females with Turner syndrome. *Reprod Biomed Online* 2009;**18**:290–5.

Leader A. Pregnancy and motherhood: the biological clock. *Sex Reprod Menopause* 2006;**4**:3–6.

Lee SJ, Shover LR, Partridge AH, *et al.* American Society of Clinical Oncology recommendations on fertility preservation in cancer patients. *J Clin Oncol* 2006;**24**(18):1–15.

Lee DR, Yang YH, Eum JH, *et al.* Effect of using slush nitrogen (SN_2) on development of microsurgically manipulated vitrified warmed mouse embryos. *Hum Reprod* 2007;**22**:2509–14.

Levi Setti PE, Albani E, Novara PV, Cesana A. Normal birth after transfer of cryopreserved human embryos generated by microinjection of cryopreserved testicular spermatozoa into cryopreserved human oocytes. *Fertil Steril* 2005;**83**(4):1041.

Levi Setti PE, Albani E, Novara PV, Cesana A, Morreale G. Cryopreservation of supernumerary oocytes in IVF/ICSI cycles. *Hum Reprod* 2006;**21**:370–5.

Li XH, Chen SU, Zhang X, *et al.* Cryopreserved oocytes of infertile couples undergoing assisted reproductive technology could be an important source of oocyte donation: a clinical report of successful pregnancies. *Hum Reprod* 2005;**20**:3390–4.

Liebermann J, Tucker MJ. Comparison of vitrification and conventional cryopreservation of day 5 and day 6 blastocysts during clinical application. *Fertil Steril* 2006;**86**(1):20–6.

Longhi A, Porcu E, Petracchi S, *et al.* Reproductive functions in female patients treated with adjuvant and neoadjuvant chemotherapy for localized osteosarcoma of the extremity. *Cancer* 2000;**89**(9):1961–5.

Lucena E, Bernal DP, Lucena C, *et al.* Successful ongoing pregnancies after vitrification of oocytes. *Fertil Steril* 2006;85:108–11.

Magistrini M, Szollosi D. Effects of cold and of isopropyl-N-phenylcarbamate on the second meiotic spindle of mouse oocytes. *Eur J Cell Biol* 1980;22(2):699–707.

Mandelbaum J, Junca AM, Plachot M, *et al.* Cryopreservation of human embryos and oocytes. *Hum Reprod* 1988a;3:117–19.

Mandelbaum J, Junca AM, Tibi C, *et al.* Cryopreservation of immature and mature hamster and human oocytes. *Ann N Y Acad Sci* 1988b;541:550–61.

Marcello MF, Nuciforo G, Romeo R, *et al.* Structural and ultrastructural study of the ovary in childhood leukemia after successful treatment. *Cancer* 1990; 66(10):2099–104.

Matorras R, Matorras F, Expósito A, Martinez L, Crisol L. Decline in human fertility rates with male age: a consequence of a decrease in male fecundity with aging? *Gynecol Obstet Invest* 2011;71(4):229–35.

Mazur P. Kinetics of water loss from cells at subzero temperatures and the likelihood of intracellular freezing. *J Gen Physiol* 1963;47:347–51.

Mazur P. Cryobiology; the freezing of biological systems. *Science* 1970;168:939–49.

Mazur P. Freezing of living cells: mechanisms and implications. *Am J Physiol* 1984;16:c125–42.

Mazur P. The freezing of living cells. *Ann N Y Acad Sci* 1988;9:514–31.

McVie JG. Cancer treatment: the last 25 years. *Cancer Treat Rev* 1999;25(6):323–31.

Meirow D. Reproduction post-chemotherapy in young cancer patients. *Mol Cell Endocrinol* 2000;169:123–31.

Meriano JS, Alexis J, Visram-Zaver S, *et al.* Tracking of oocyte dysmorphisms for ICSI patients may prove relevant to the outcome in subsequent patient cycle. *Hum Reprod* 2001;16:2118–23.

Mhatre P, Mhatre J. Orthotopic ovarian transplant–review and three surgical techniques. *Pediatr Transplant* 2006;10:782–7.

Miller KA, Elkind-Hirsch K, Levy B, *et al.* Pregnancy after cryopreservation of donor oocytes and preimplantation genetic diagnosis of embryos in a patient with ovarian failure. *Fertil Steril* 2004;82:211–14.

Montag M, van der Ven K, Dorn C, *et al.* Birth after double cryopreservation of human oocytes at metaphase II and pronuclear stages. *Fertil Steril* 2006;85:751.e5–e7.

Nawroth F, Kissing K. Pregnancy after intracytoplasmatic sperm injection (ICSI) of cryopreserved human oocytes. *Acta Obstet Gynecol Scand* 1998;77:462–3.

Newton CR, Fisher J, Feyles V, *et al.* Changes in patient preferences in the disposal of cryopreserved embryos. *Hum Reprod* 2007;22(12):3124–8.

Nicosia SV, Matus-Ridley M, Meadows AT. Gonadal effects of cancer therapy in girls. *Cancer* 1985;55(10):2364–72.

Nielsen J, Sillesen I, Hansen KB. Fertility in women with Turner's syndrome. Case report and review of literature. *Br J Obstet Gynaecol* 1979;86:833–5.

Nieto Y, Cagnoni PJ, Shpall EJ, *et al.* A predictive model for relapse in high-risk primary breast cancer patients treated with high-dose chemotherapy and autologous stem-cell transplant. *Clin Cancer Res* 1999;5(11): 3425–31.

Nikolaou D, Templeton A. Early ovarian ageing: a hypothesis – detection and clinical relevance. *Hum Reprod* 2003;18:1137–9

Notrica J, Kanzepolsky L, Divita A, Neuspiller F, Polak de Fried E. A healthy female born after ICSI of a cryopreserved oocyte and cryopreserved spermatozoa banked prior to radiotherapy in a patient with a seminoma: a case report. *Fertil Steril* 2003; 80(Suppl 3):S149.

Nottola SA, Macchiarelli G, Coticchio G, *et al.* Ultrastructure of human oocytes after slow cooling cryopreservation using different sucrose concentrations. *Hum Reprod* 2007; 22(4):1123–33.

Nottola SA, Coticchio G, De Santis L, *et al.* Ultrastructure of human mature oocytes after slow freezing cryopreservation using ethylene glycol. *Reprod Biomed Online* 2008;17(3):368–77.

Noyes N, Chang C, Liu H, *et al.* Presence of meiotic spindle predicts embryo competence following oocyte cryopreservation. *Fertil Steril* 2006;**86**:S2.

Noyes N, Porcu E, Borini A. Over 900 oocyte cryopreservation babies born with no apparent increase in congenital anomalies. *Reprod Biomed Online* 2009;**18**(6):769–76.

Okimura T, Kato K, Zhan Q, *et al.* Update on clinical efficiency of the vitrification method for human oocytes in an in vitro fertilization program. *Fertil Steril* 2005;**84**(Suppl 1):S174.

Oktay K. Further evidence on the safety and success of ovarian stimulation with letrozole and tamoxifen in breast cancer patients undergoing in vitro fertilization to cryopreserve their embryos for fertility preservation. *Clin Oncol* 2005;**23**(16):3858–9.

Oktay K, Sonmezer M. Ovarian tissue banking for cancer patients: fertility preservation, not just ovarian cryopreservation. *Hum Reprod* 2004;**19**(3):477–80.

Oktay K, Hourvitz A, Sahin G, *et al.* Letrozole reduces estrogen and gonadotropin exposure in women with breast cancer undergoing ovarian stimulation before chemotherapy. *J Clin Endocrinol Metab* 2006;**91**(10):3885–90.

Oktay K, Demirtas E, Son WY, *et al.* In vitro maturation of germinal vesicle oocytes recovered after premature luteinizing hormone surge: description of a novel approach to fertility preservation. *Fertil Steril* 2008;**89**:228.e19–22.

Oktay K, Rodriguez-Wallberg KA, Sahin G. Fertility preservation by ovarian stimulation and oocyte cryopreservation in a 14-year-old adolescent with Turner syndrome mosaicism and impending premature ovarian failure. *Fertil Steril* 2010;**94**:753.e15–19.

Oldenbourg R. A new view on polarization microscopy. *Nature* 1996;**381**:811–12.

Pal L, Leykin L, Schifren JL, *et al.* Malignancy may adversely influence the quality and behaviour of oocytes. *Hum Reprod* 1998;**13**(7):1837–40.

Park CW, Yang KM, Kim HO, *et al.* Outcomes of controlled ovarian hyperstimulation/in vitro fertilization for infertile patients with borderline ovarian tumor after conservative treatment. *J Korean Med Sci.* 2007;**22** (Suppl):S134–8.

Park SE, Son WY, Lee SH, *et al..* Chromosome and spindle configurations of human oocytes matured in vitro after cryopreservation at the germinal vesicle stage. *Fertil Steril* 1997; **68**(5):920–6.

Parkening TA, Tsunoda Y, Chang MC. Effects of various low temperatures, cryoprotective agents and cooling rates on the survival, fertilizability and development of frozen–thawed mouse eggs. *J Exp Zool* 1976;**197**(3):369–74.

Parmegiani L, Cogniti GE, Bernardi S, *et al.* Freezing within 2 h from oocyte retrieval increases the efficiency of human oocyte cryopreservation when using a slow freezing/rapid thawing protocol with high sucrose concentration. *Hum Reprod* 2008;**12**:1–7.

Pasquino AM, Passeri F, Pucarelli I, Segni M, Municchi G. Spontaneous pubertal development in Turner's syndrome. Italian Study Group for Turner's syndrome. *J Clin Endocrinol Metab* 1997;**82**(6):1810–13.

Paynter SJ, Borini A, Bianchi V, *et al.* Volume changes of mature human oocytes on exposure to cryoprotectant solution used in slow cooling procedures. *Hum Reprod* 2005;**20**(5):1194–9.

Pelletier C, Keefe DL, Trimarchi JR. Noninvasive polarized light microscopy quantitatively distinguishes the multilaminar structure of the zona pellucida of living human eggs and embryos. *Fertil Steril* 2004;**81**(Suppl 1):850–6.

Pennings G. The validity of contracts to dispose of frozen embryos. *J Med Ethics* 2002;**28**:295–8.

Pensis M, Loumaye E, Psalti I. Screening of conditions for rapid freezing of human oocytes: preliminary study toward their cryopreservation. *Fertil Steril* 1989;**52**:787–94.

Pickering SJ, Johnson MH. The influence of cooling on the organization of the meiotic spindle of the mouse oocyte. *Hum Reprod* 1987;**2**(3):207–16.

Pickering SJ, Braude PR, Johnson MH, Cant A, Currie J. Transient cooling to room temperature can cause irreversible disruption to the meiotic spindle in human oocytes. *Fertil Steril* 1990;**54**:102–8.

Pinto AB, Gopal M, Herzog TJ, Pfeifer JD, Williams DB. Successful in vitro fertilization pregnancy after conservative management of endometrial cancer. *Fertil Steril* 2001;**76**(4):826–9.

Polak de Fried E, Notrica J, Rubinstein M, Marazzi A, Gómez Gonzalez M. Pregnancy after human donor oocyte cryopreservation and thawing in association with intracytoplasmic sperm injection in a patient with ovarian failure. *Fertil Steril* 1998;**69**:555–7.

Porcu E. Cryopreservation of oocytes: indications, risks and outcomes. *Hum Reprod* 2005;**20**(Suppl 1):50.

Porcu E, Fabbri R, Seracchioli R, *et al.* Birth of a healthy female after intracytoplasmic sperm injection of cryopreserved human oocytes. *Fertil Steril* 1997;**68**:724–6.

Porcu E, Fabbri R, Seracchioli R, *et al.* Birth of six healthy children after intracytoplasmic sperm injection of cryopreserved human oocytes. *Hum Reprod* 1998;**13**:124.

Porcu E, Fabbri R, Ciotti PM, *et al.* Ongoing pregnancy after intracytoplasmic sperm injection of epididymal spermatozoa into cryopreserved human oocytes. *J Assist Reprod Genet* 1999a;**16**:283–5.

Porcu E, Fabbri R, Petracchi S, Ciotti PM, Flamingni C. Ongoing pregnancy after intracytoplasmic injection of testicular spermatozoa into cryopreserved human oocytes. *Am J Obstet Gynecol* 1999b;**180**:1044–5.

Porcu E, Fabbri R, Marsella T, *et al.* Clinical experience and application of oocyte cryopreservation. *Mol Cell Endocrinol* 2000a;**169**:33–7.

Porcu E, Fabbri R, Seracchioli R, *et al.* Obstetric, perinatal outcome and follow up of children conceived from cryopreserved oocytes. *Fertil Steril* 2000b;**74**(Suppl 1):S48.

Porcu E, Fabbri R, Ciotti P, *et al.* Four healthy children from frozen human oocytes and frozen human sperms. *Fertil Steril* 2001;**76**(Suppl 1):S76.

Porcu E, Fabbri R, Ciotti P, *et al.* Oocytes or embryo storage. *Fertil Steril* 2002; **78**(Suppl 1):S15.

Porcu E, Fabbri R, Damiano G, *et al.* Oocyte cryopreservation in oncological patients.

Eur J Obstet Gynecol Reprod Biol 2004;**113**(Suppl 1):S14–16.

Porcu E, Venturoli S, Damiano G, *et al.* Healthy twins delivered after oocyte cryopreservation and bilateral ovariectomy for ovarian cancer. *Reprod Biomed Online* 2008;**17**:267–9.

Purushothaman R, Lazareva O, Oktay K, Ten S. Markers of ovarian reserve in young girls with Turner's syndrome. *Fertil Steril* 2010;**94**(4):1557–9.

Quintans CJ, Donaldson MJ, Bertolino MV, Godoy H, Pasqualini RS. Birth of a healthy baby after transfer of embryos that were cryopreserved for 8.9 years. *Fertil Steril* 2002;**77**(5):1074–6.

Rall WF, Fahy GM. Ice-free cryopreservation of mouse embryos at −196 degrees C by vitrification. *Nature* 1985;**313**:573–5.

Renard JP, Babinet C. High survival of mouse embryos after rapid freezing and thawing inside plastic straws with 1,2 propanediol as cryoprotectant. *J Exp Zool* 1984;**230**(3):443–8.

Requena A, Herrero J, Landeras J, *et al.* Use of letrozole in assisted reproduction: a systematic review and meta-analysis. *Hum Reprod Update* 2008;**14**:571–82.

Rienzi L, Martinez F, Ubaldi F, *et al.* Polscope analysis of meiotic spindle changes in living metaphase II human oocytes during the freezing and thawing procedures. *Hum Reprod* 2004;**19**:655–9.

Risco R, Elmoazzen H, Doughty M, Xiaoming H, Toner M. Thermal performance of quartz capillary for vitrification. *Cryobiology* 2007;**55**:222–9.

Ruvalcaba L, Marínez R, Cuneo S, *et al.* Improving donor programs with an oocyte bank using vitrification. *Fertil Steril* 2005; **84**(Suppl 1):S70.

Sànchez-Serrano M, Crespo J, Mirabet V, *et al.* Twins born after transplantation of ovarian cortical tissue and oocyte vitrification. *Fertil Steril* 2010;**93**:268.e11–13.

Sathananthan AH, Trounson A, Freemann L, Brady T. The effects of cooling human oocytes. *Hum Reprod* 1988;**3**:968–77.

Selman H, Angelini A, Barnocchi N, *et al.* Ongoing pregnancies after vitrification of human oocytes using a combined solution of ethylene glycol and dimethyl sulfoxide. *Fertil Steril* 2006;**86**:997–1000.

Sherman JK. Temperature shock and cold-storage of unfertilized mouse eggs. *Fertil Steril* 1959;**10**:384–96.

Sherman JK, Lin TP. Effect of glycerol and low temperature on survival of unfertilized mouse eggs. *Nature* 1958;**181**:785–6.

Smith GD, Fioravanti J, Hassun PA, *et al.* Prospective randomized controlled study of human oocyte cryopreservation by slow-rate freezing and/or vitrification. *Fertil Steril* 2006;**86**(Suppl 2):S96.

Smith GD, Serafini PC, Fioravanti J, *et al.* Prospective randomized comparison of human oocyte cryopreservation with slow-rate freezing or vitrification. *Fertil Steril* 2010;**94**(6):2088–95.

Smitz JEJ, Thompson JG, Gilchrist RB. The promise of in vitro maturation in assisted reproduction and fertility preservation. *Semin Reprod Med* 2011;**29**(1):24–37.

Son WY, Park SE, Lee KA, *et al.* Effects of 1,2-propanediol and freezing on the in vitro developmental capacity of human immature oocytes. *Fertil Steril* 1996;**66**:996–9.

Stoop D, Nekkebroeck J, Devroey P. A survey on the intentions and attitudes towards oocyte cryopreservation for non-medical reasons among women of reproductive age. *Hum Reprod* 2011;**26**(3):655–61.

Stachecki JJ, Cohen J, Willadsen S. Detrimental effects of sodium during mouse oocyte cryopreservation. *Biol Reprod* 1998;**59**:395–400.

Swapp GH, Johnston AW, Watt JL, Couzin DA, Stephen GS. A fertile woman with non-mosaic Turner's syndrome. Case report and review of the literature. *J Obstet Gynaecol* 1989;**96**(7):876–80.

Tarani L, Lampariello S, Raguso G, *et al.* Pregnancy in patients with Turner's syndrome: six new cases and review of literature. *Gynecol Endocrinol* 1998;**12**:83–7.

The Ethics Committee of the American Society for Reproductive Medicine. Fertility preservation and reproduction in cancer patients. *Fertil Steril* 2005;**83**(6):1622–8.

Tjer GC, Chiu TT, Cheung LP, Lok IH, Haines CJ. Birth of a healthy baby after transfer of blastocysts derived from cryopreserved human oocytes fertilized with frozen spermatozoa. *Fertil Steril* 2005;**83**:1547–9.

Toth TL, Baka SG, Veeck LL, *et al.* Fertilization and in vitro development of cryopreserved human prophase I oocytes. *Fertil Steril* 1994;**61**:891–4.

Trounson A. Preservation of human eggs and embryos. *Fertil Steril* 1986;**46**:1–12.

Trounson A, Mohr L. Human pregnancy following cryopreservation, thawing and transfer of an eight-cell embryo. *Nature* 1983;**305**:707–9.

Tucker M, Wright G, Morton P, *et al.* Preliminary experience with human oocyte cryopreservation using 1,2-propanediol and sucrose. *Hum Reprod* 1996;**11**:1513–15.

Tucker MJ, Wright G, Morton PC, Massey JB. Birth after cryopreservation of immature oocytes with subsequent in vitro maturation. *Fertil Steril* 1998a;**70**:578–9.

Tucker MJ, Morton PC, Wright G, Sweitzer CL, Massey JB. Clinical application of human egg cryopreservation. *Hum Reprod* 1998b;**13**(11):3156–9.

UK Office for the National Statistics. Who is having babies? *Office for National Statistics Statistical Bulletin* 2008:1–11.

Van Blerkom J, Davis PW. Cytogenetic, cellular, and developmental consequences of cryopreservation of immature and mature mouse and human oocytes. *Microsc Res Tech* 1994;**27**:165–93.

Van Der Elst J, Van Den Abbeel E, Nerinckx S, Van Steirteghem A. A parthenogenetic activation pattern and microtubular organization of the mouse oocyte after exposure to 1,2-propanediol. *Cryobiology* 1992;**29**:549–62.

Van Uem JF, Siebzehnrubl ER, Schuh B, *et al.* Birth after cryopreservation of unfertilised oocytes. *Lancet* 1987;**1**:752–3.

Vincent C, Garnier V, Heyman Y, Renard JP. Solvent effects on cytoskeletal organization and in-vivo survival after freezing of rabbit oocytes. *J Reprod Fertil* 1989;**87**:809–20.

Virant-Klun I, Bacer-Kermavner LB, Tomazevic T, Vrtacnik-Bokal E. Slow oocyte freezing and thawing in couples with no sperm or an insufficient number of sperm on the day of in vitro fertilization. *Reprod Biol Endocrinol* 2011;9:19.

Wallace WH, Anderson RA, Irvine DS. Fertility preservation for young patiens with cancer: who is at risk and what can be offered? *Lancet Oncol* 2005;6:209–18.

Wang WH, Meng L, Hackett RJ, Oldenbourg R, Keefe DL. Limited recovery of meiotic spindles in living human oocytes after cooling-rewarming observed using polarized light microscopy. *Hum Reprod* 2001;16:2374–8.

Wennerholm UB, Söderström-Anttila V, Bergh C, *et al.* Children born after cryopreservation of embryos or oocytes: a systematic review of outcome data. *Hum Reprod* 2009;24(9):2158–72.

Whittingham DG. Fertilization in vitro and development to term of unfertilized mouse oocytes previously stored at −196 degrees C. *J Reprod Fertil* 1977;49:89–94.

Whittingham DG, Leibo SP, Mazur P. Survival of mouse embryos frozen to −196 degrees and −269 degrees C. *Science* 1972;178:411–14.

Winslow K, Yang D, Blohm P, *et al.* Oocyte cryopreservation /a three year follow up of sixteen births. *Fertil Steril* 2001;76(Suppl 1):S120–1.

Wu J, Zhang L, Wang X. In vitro maturation, fertilization and embryo development after ultrarapid freezing of immature human oocytes. *Reproduction* 2001;121:389–93.

Wurfel W, Schleyer M, Krusmann G, Hertwig IV, Fiedler K. Fertilization of cryopreserved and thawed human oocytes (Cryo-Oo) by injection of spermatozoa (ICSI)–medical management of sterility and case report of a twin pregnancy. *Zentralbl Gynakol* 1999;121:444–8.

Yang D, Blohm P, Winslow K, Cramer L. A twin pregnancy after microinjection of human cryopreserved oocyte with a specially developed oocyte cryopreservation regime. *Fertil Steril* 1998;70(Suppl 1):S239.

Yang D, Winslow K, Blohm P, *et al.* Oocyte donation using cryopreserved donor oocytes. *Fertil Steril* 2002;78(Suppl 1):S14.

Yang D, Brown SE, Nguyen K, *et al.* Live birth after the transfer of human embryos developed from cryopreserved oocytes harvested before cancer treatment. *Fertil Steril* 2007;87:1469.e1–4.

Yarali H, Bozdag G, Aksu T, Ayhan A. A successful pregnancy after intracytoplasmic sperm injection and embryo transfer in a patient with endometrial cancer who was treated conservatively. *Fertil Steril* 2004;81(1):214–16.

Yaron Y, Ochshorn Y, Amit A, *et al.* Patients with Turner's syndrome may have an inherent endometrial abnormality affecting receptivity in oocyte donation. *Fertil Steril* 1996;65:1249–52.

Yoon TK, Kim TJ, Park SE, *et al.* Live births after vitrification of oocytes in a stimulated in vitro fertilization-embryo transfer program. *Fertil Steril* 2003;79:1323–6.

Yoon TK, Lee DR, Cha SK, *et al.* Survival rate of human oocytes and pregnancy outcome after vitrification using slush nitrogen in assisted reproductive technologies. *Fertil Steril* 2007;88:925–6.

Young E, Kenny A, Puigdomenech E, *et al.* Triplet pregnancy after intracytoplasmic sperm injection of cryopreserved oocytes: case report. *Fertil Steril* 1998;70:360–1.

Index

Figures and tables appear in bold typeface.

Printed in the United States
by Baker & Taylor Publisher Services